CLINICAL APPROACHES TO FAMILY VIOLENCE

James C. Hansen, Editor
Laurence R. Barnhill, Volume Editor

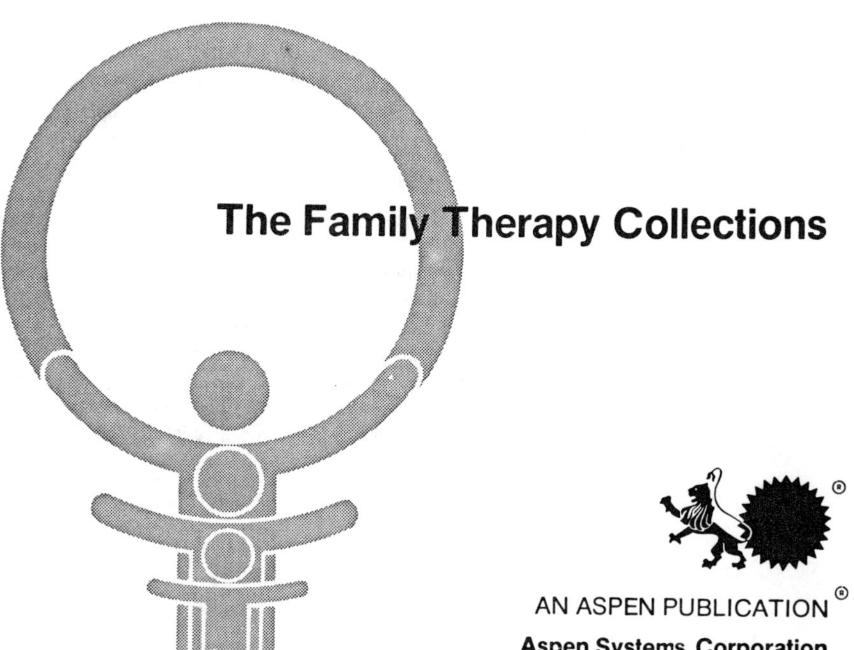

The Family Therapy Collections

AN ASPEN PUBLICATION®

Aspen Systems Corporation
Rockville, Maryland
London
1982

Library of Congress Cataloging in Publication Data
Main entry under title:

Clinical approaches to family violence.

(The Family therapy collections)
Includes bibliographical references.
1. Family violence—Psychological aspects.
2. Mentally ill—Family relationships.
3. Family psychotherapy.
I. Barnhill, Laurence R.   II. Series.   [DNLM: 1. Family.
2. Violence.   3. Family therapy.   BF 575.A3 C641]
RC569.5.F3C57   1982   616.85'82   82-11444
ISBN 0-89443-804-2

Publisher: John Marozsan
Managing Editor: Margot Raphael
Printing and Manufacturing: Debbie Collins

Library of Congress Catalog Card Number: 82-11444
ISBN: 0-89443-804-2

Printed in the United States of America

1 2 3 4 5

Table of Contents

Board of Editors

Board of Editors
(continued)

Contributors

Volume Editor

LAURENCE R. BARNHILL, PH.D.
Coordinator
Outpatient and Emergency Services
South Central Community Mental Health Center
Bloomington, Indiana

RICHARD C. BEDROSIAN
Director
Massachusetts Center for
Cognitive Therapy
Westmeadow Medical Center
Westboro, Massachusetts

HERB GOLDBERG
Licensed Psychologist
Los Angeles, California

GWEN BERGHORN
Supervisor
Child Abuse Service
Director Unified Services Project
South Central Community Mental
Health Center
Bloomington, Indiana

BLAIR JUSTICE
Professor of Psychology
Behavioral Sciences
University of Texas School of
Public Health
Houston, Texas

FRANK A. ELLIOTT
Emeritus Professor, Neurology
University of Pennsylvania
Medical School
Philadelphia, Pennsylvania
Consultant
Pennsylvania Hospital
Philadelphia, Pennsylvania

RITA JUSTICE
Psychologist
Houston, Texas

DENIS J. MADDEN
Director
Clinical Research Program for
Violent Behavior
Assistant Professor
Department of Psychiatry
University of Maryland School of
Medicine
Baltimore, Maryland

GORDON GIBSON
Director of Evaluation Research
South Central Community Mental
Health Center
Bloomington, Indiana

Contributors
(continued)

RODNEY J. SHAPIRO
Director
Family Therapy Program
Veterans Administration Medical
Center
San Francisco, California

MARGARET F. SQUIRES
Addictions Therapist
South Central Community Mental
Health Center
Bloomington, Indiana

ANTHONY SIRACUSA
Clinical Team Leader
Child Abuse Service
South Central Community Mental
Health Center
Bloomington, Indiana

M. ELLEN TRAICOFF
Administrator/Clinical Supervisor
Family Violence
Southlake Center for Mental
Health
Merriville, Indiana

Preface

THE FAMILY THERAPY COLLECTIONS IS A SERIAL PUB-
lication that reviews topics of current interest to practicing professionals
in the mental health field. Each volume provides in-depth coverage of a
single significant aspect of family therapy, with emphasis on translating
theory and research into practical applications.

This volume of *The Family Therapy Collections* focuses on clinical
approaches to violence that occurs within the family. Despite the growing
body of information about the causes of violent behavior and methods of
intervention, mental health professionals have been slow to respond to the
needs of these clients. Family therapists need to be aware that violence
occurs more frequently in families with mental health problems than is
reported. Individuals or families who enter therapy may not report the
violent incidents, either because they fear reprisals or they do not see that
the violence is relevant to their problems.

The early research in this field concentrated on child abuse and attributed violence to individual personal problems. Although this view leads
to therapeutic intervention, treatment focuses on only one family member. Recognition of the multidimensional aspects of violence in the family clearly broadens the scope of appropriate intervention.

This volume presents a broad overview of violence in the family—
including child abuse, adolescent abuse, and marital violence—and also
provides information on the effects of alcoholism and neurological conditions that may be involved. Armed with a more comprehensive knowledge of violence in the family setting, a therapist is better prepared to
intervene.

It seems appropriate for family therapists to play a key role in meeting the needs for intervention in these families. The treatment of violence in family units is an area undergoing development, and modifications in family therapy concepts and strategies are necessary. The treatment of family violence is a particularly difficult undertaking for the therapist who is working alone. Authors in this volume illustrate methods of working with couples and with the whole family, and suggest the need for professional and interagency support and cooperation in these cases.

Laurence Barnhill, Ph.D., is the Volume Editor. Dr. Barnhill is adjunct faculty in the Department of Psychology at Indiana University and Coordinator of Outpatient and Emergency Services at South Central Community Mental Health Center in Bloomington, Indiana. There he has developed a child abuse service, organized a group treatment program for violent men, acted as a consultant for the women's shelter and for the youth shelter's therapy program for adolescents in crisis, and testified before the state legislature on domestic violence legislation. He also is Director of the Bloomington Family Institute, which offers a program of professional training and family life education.

The author of numerous articles on family therapy and family violence, he has also presented papers and workshops on violence and family therapy. Dr. Barnhill's expertise in these areas makes him well qualified to edit this volume. He has identified leaders in this field who have provided a collection of articles that will serve as an excellent resource of practical information and effective approaches for the professional therapist.

James C. Hansen
Editor
August 1982

Introduction

THE LAST DECADE HAS SHOWN AN UPSURGE OF INTEREST in addressing the problem of violence in the family on the part of many professions, including medicine, law, mental health, sociology, government, and others. Some efforts are under way to organize and integrate the knowledge base developing in the new field. Most emphasize theoretical or sociological research; a few mix theoretical approaches with clinical material. This volume represents an effort to go beyond the general overview approach and to provide specific suggestions for practicing clinicians on practical approaches to treating intrafamilial violence.

Current examples of demonstrable successes in dealing with this problem are presented here. The authors are experienced practitioners who share their difficulties as well as their creative solutions in developing clinical and programmatic strategies that are really working. Implicit in this emphasis on innovation is the conclusion that traditional modes of treatment have not been effective with this problem.

What modifications in traditional approaches to therapy are necessary for effective treatment of intrafamilial violence? Family-oriented clinicians have an advantage here, in that it seems obvious to them (and to some others as well) that treatment must focus on the family. However, while a family perspective must be maintained, the usual family therapy format of sitting down with the whole family together is often not possible or not effective, and thus must be modified in accordance with the situation.

In addition to a family-oriented but flexible approach, a second requirement is a capability for crisis intervention. This is necessary because so many of these cases present in crisis or go into crisis during treatment. A third requirement in clinical work with family violence is an assessment of the etiology of the violence—there can be many causes and some are more obvious than others. The theme of several articles, in fact, is etiological factors in family violence, and several others emphasize the relevance of the issues to treatment.

A fourth requirement in treating these clients is the ability to deal with the generally high level of resistance of these families to treatment. Many are coerced into treatment, whether at the insistence of family members or by the order of a court. Drs. Blair and Rita Justice attempt to dispel the myth that coercive treatment does not work—a theme also discussed by Shapiro, Traicoff, and Berghorn and Siracusa.

A fifth area important to many of these authors is the need for support for the clinicians involved in these cases. This support can be practical, including protective shelters for clients, court orders necessary to keep the families in treatment, or additional resources such as detoxification facilities. The support can also be more personal, since the impact of these cases on the therapist can be so intense, as discussed by Shapiro, Madden, Berghorn and Siracusa, and Bedrosian.

Since so many factors are involved in the treatment of clients in the setting of intrafamilial violence, we can appreciate the diversity of approaches the authors use to delineate effective clinical styles and combinations of techniques that have proven most effective. The first papers address etiological factors in family violence. Drs. Blair and Rita Justice are well-known leaders in the area and present their cogent perspective on the etiology of child abuse as well as specifically addressing the issue of coerced treatment. They discuss the key question of why stress leads to violence rather than to other symptoms in these families, and detail a clear and practical treatment strategy. Dr. Herb Goldberg (author of *The Hazards of Being Male,* 1976, and co-author of *Creative Aggression,* 1974) focuses on the affect involved in spouse- abuse as well as the questions of socialization and sex-role stereotypes that are often involved in that problem. Dr. Frank Elliott, distinguished Emeritus Professor of Neurology of the University of Pennsylvania Medical School, offers the medical perspective so often ignored by nonphysicians. His overview includes neurological and metabolic problems associated with violence, presents information on distinguishing between medical and personality abnormalities, and suggests some considerations for medical and psycho-therapeutic treatment.

The extent and seriousness of the problem of violence are documented in a clinical epidemiology study by Barnhill, Squires, and Gibson. They detail the amount, types, and levels of violence in a clinic population and confirm earlier work indicating that the vast majority of violent incidents occur within families.

The next three papers focus on special populations involved in violence. Dr. Rodney Shapiro, Director of the Family Therapy Program at the Veterans Administration Medical Center in San Francisco, discusses the relationship of alcoholism to family violence. He points out the fascinating parallels between the two areas of study: both are conceptually complex—involving social, behavioral, and medical factors—both problems are known to be difficult to treat, and they often coexist. Dr. Shapiro takes a broad view, encompassing the complexities of etiology, phases of treatment, resistance, and countertransference, and yet makes the area seem manageable and easily comprehensible. Adolescent violence is an important but less frequently discussed issue of family violence. The family dynamics involved and treatment considerations are discussed by Dr. Denis Madden, the Director of the Clinical Research Program for Violent Behavior at the University of Maryland School of Medicine in Baltimore. Ellen Traicoff developed and supervises the first CMHC based women's shelter. As both a women's advocate and trained family therapist, she presents a systems perspective on the use of shelters in family treatment.

Looking toward the innovations of the future, Dr. Richard Bedrosian, Director of the Massachusetts Center for Cognitive Therapy, discusses a new clinical approach that shows considerable promise in treating family violence. He combines practical techniques from strategic family therapy and cognitive-behavioral schools of thought to form a pragmatic and efficient new synthesis. Gwen Berghorn, Project Director of the federally funded demonstration Unified Services Project, and Anthony Siracusa, supervisor of a child abuse treatment team, broaden our clinical view to include the community context. They present practical steps for team building and agency training as well as suggestions on involving the community at large in the treatment of family violence.

Important advances are being made in the treatment of clients involved in intrafamilial violence. Successful approaches are in use and can be documented. Innovative and practical new concepts and intervention strategies and widespread use of the tools of psychological, interpersonal, medical, and community organization professionals hold considerable promise for more comprehensive and effective interventions with these families.

Acknowledgments

I would like to acknowledge the influence of Dr. John R. Lion, Professor of Psychiatry, University of Maryland Medical Center at Baltimore, on my research and clinical work with the problem of violence. His clear and precise research and scientific writing on the problem of violence, beginning in 1972, together with his emphasis on practical effectiveness in clinical practice, have been and remain a model and an inspiration. As always, the support of my wife Kristine made the project possible and worthwhile.

REFERENCES

Bach, G., & Goldberg, H. *Creative aggression.* New York: Avon, 1974.
Goldberg, H. *The hazards of being male.* New York: New American Library, 1976.
Lion, J. *Evaluation and management of the violent patient.* Springfield, Ill.: Charles C Thomas, 1972.

Laurence R. Barnhill
Volume Editor
August 1982

1. Etiology of Physical Abuse of Children and Dynamics of Coercive Treatment

Blair Justice, Ph.D.
Professor of Psychology
University of Texas School of Public Health
Houston, Texas

Rita Justice, Ph.D.
Psychologist in Private Practice
Houston, Texas

One

"THE PATIENT HAS TO WANT TO BE IN TREATMENT FOR THERE to be any lasting changes." That sentence sums up the traditional position held by many therapists. Therapeutic outcome has been thought to be a function, in part at least, of a client's willingness to receive treatment. In actual fact, there is woefully little documentation of the effect of "coercive" therapy, such as that ordered by courts referring patients for treatment. One recent study that did examine the difference in compliance and outcome in the treatment of self-referred versus court-referred sexual offenders found no significant differences in treatment results between the two groups (Maletzky, 1980). Findings indicated that the same techniques successfully applied to voluntary patients with maladaptive sexual approach behaviors can be applied effectively to an involuntary population as well.

In working with child-abusing families since 1973, our experience has been that significant, lasting changes can be brought about even if the clients come into treatment under coercion (Justice & Justice, 1976, 1979). Between 1973 and 1979, the parents in 40 families in which there had been physical abuse of children completed therapy with us. All these couples were referred by child protective agencies in our area, primarily the Harris County Child Welfare Unit. In 75% of the cases, there had been a court order removing the couple's child from the home. The parents were given to understand that their chances of getting the child back would be greatly enhanced if they underwent therapy. In the other 25%, parents were told that they would much more likely be allowed to keep their child at home with them if they went into therapy. Thus, when most of the couples entered treatment, they came with resentment—resentment at having been told, in effect, that they had to come. We are convinced that most, if not all, the couples we treated would not have entered therapy if they had not been told to do so.

Among those 40 couples, there has been one reported case of recurrence of abuse. This is not to say that every couple sent by the courts for therapy had a successful outcome. Six couples dropped out of therapy and subsequently lost custody of their children. Even so, the proportion of those who did have a successful outcome supports the fact that people do change even if initially forced into therapy. Without coercion, most physically abusive families would not undergo treatment. And without treatment, the children in the family continue to be at risk of being abused.

Clearly, people are not going to change quickly and easily if they are extremely resistant, but they are unlikely to change at all if they are not put into a position that makes change at least possible. The probability of physically abusive parents becoming competent caretakers of their children without professional treatment is extremely low. Even lower are the odds that these parents would voluntarily reach out for help. Almost every abusive parent we have worked with was physically and/or emotionally abused as a child. This has been true of both the parent who actually inflicts the physical injury and the passive spouse. Such individuals learned to be distrustful early in life, and they carry that distrust into adulthood. People have failed them so often that they have long since ceased to expect any positive outcomes from their encounters with others. This mistrust overrides any impulse to ask for help. So, unless they are forced into getting help, abusive parents are not likely to seek it.

Significantly, most abusive parents *do* keep coming to therapy when ordered to do so, and they do change. They come because their children matter to them and they want them back. The fact that the parents change and that their changes endure supports the behavior therapy theory that if people will practice a new behavior, whether they want to or not, that behavior will be adopted, and feelings will change in a positive direction. As noted by Burns (1980):

> You can substantially change the way you feel by changing the way you act . . . .Your error is your belief that motivation comes first, and then leads to activation and success. But it is usually the other way around; action must come first, and the motivation comes later on. (p.118)

Effecting change is of the utmost urgency because of the seriousness of the problem. The physical abuse of children is a major public health problem. Kempe (1971) reported that approximately 25% of all fractures seen in the first two years of life and 10% to 15% of all trauma seen in the first three years are due to abuse by parents or parent surrogates. The true prevalence of physical child abuse is difficult to determine, but estimates of the total number of actual cases per year range from 2.5 million to 41.1 million. Most recently Straus, Gelles, and Steinmetz (1979), on the basis of a nationally representative sample, reported 14.2 cases per 100 families. In Harris County, Texas, where we have worked, the number of physically abused children investigated by the child welfare unit is 450 *per month.*

Why Child Abuse Happens

What distinguishes the abusing family from the nonabusing one? The vast majority of people who have physically abused their children are not maniacs or even parents who do not love their children. A very small percentage are psychotic. As a group, they defy psychiatric classification. They come from all socioeconomic groups and all educational levels. How then do they differ from parents who do not abuse?

One possible answer is suggested by the environmental stress theorists, as represented by Gil (1970). In his nationwide case-register study, Gil found that reports of child abuse were heavily concentrated among the poor. Child abuse, he suggested, may be regarded largely as being one more aspect of the poverty syndrome. In Gil's words (1969):

> Life in poverty generates many additional stressful experiences which are likely to become precipitating factors in child abuse. The poor are subject to the same psychological conditions which may cause violent behavior toward children as are the non-poor; but in addition to this, they are subject to the special environmental distresses and strains associated with the socio-economic deprivation. (p. 862)

A similar viewpoint is present in Gelles's social-psychological theory of child abuse. Essentially, Gelles (1973) sees child abuse as a particular form of adaptation to stress. He also considers such factors as societal values and norms, socialization experience, and ''psychopathic states.''

But he emphasizes such stress areas as socioeconomic position of parents, marital stresses, excessive number of children, unemployment, social isolation, unwanted or "problem" children, and immediate precipitating situations such as an argument or child misbehavior.

Probably the foremost theory in the field of child abuse is the psychodynamic theory developed by Kempe, Helfer, and their colleagues (1972). This approach presents a three-factor theory: First, the parents must have the potential to abuse, primarily as a result of receiving an inadequate "mothering imprint" in their own childhoods. Second, the child must be seen by the parent as being "special" or different, whether he or she really is or not. Third, a crisis must occur that triggers the abuse.

While all these psychodynamic theories of child abuse recognize stress as playing a part, primarily as a precipitating event, our focus is on the particular role of stress from life change events. The study of change events dates back to Meyer's work in the first quarter of this century. For each of his patients he had what he called a "life chart," on which he recorded "changes of habitat," school entrance, graduations, various jobs, dates of births and deaths in the family, and other events. He proceeded to chart these events against changes in physical or mental health. Meyer saw that any change, good or bad, required adaptation and was, therefore, stressful.

Holmes and Rahe (1967) picked up on Meyer's work in describing the influence of life change events on the onset of illness. The Social Readjustment Rating Scale came out of this work. This scale lists 43 events requiring readjustment by a person experiencing them. The events were assigned a numerical value that represents the estimated amount of adjustment required for each event.

To assess how stress from change events and other factors may be associated with child abuse, we administered a questionnaire to two groups of parents. The questionnaire included 39 questions plus the Schedule of Recent Experiences. The first group was made up of 35 parents who had abused their children. The second group contained 35 parents—matched in age, education, and economic status to the abusing parents. The second group had no record of having abused their children but had experienced various other difficulties with them. Both groups of parents included a cross section of socioeconomic classes, weighted toward the lower-middle and working class.

Table 1-1 Distribution of Life-Change Scores for Abusing and Nonabusing Parents

Parent group	Life-change scores			
	No crisis 0–149	Mild crisis 150–199	Moderate crisis 200–299	Major crisis 300+
Abusers (N = 35) $\overline{X}$ = 233.63	4	9	14	8
Nonabusers (N = 35) $\overline{X}$ = 123.62	25	5	3	2

[a]x^2 = 25.69, p < .001; [t]ind = 4.28, p < .001.

Source: Justice, B., and Justice, R. *The Abusing Family.* New York: Human Sciences Press, 1976, p. 29.

The most significant difference between the abusing and nonabusing parents emerged on the Schedule of Recent Experiences, depicting life events for the two groups during the 12 months preceding problems with their children. As can be seen in Table 1-1, the abusing parents had much higher life change scores. Their lives were in a chronic state of what Holmes and Rahe call a "life crisis." The mean score on the rating scale was 234 for the abusing parents and 124 for the nonabusing group (Justice & Justice, 1976). Scores of 150 to 199 are classified as constituting a mild life crisis, 200 to 299 as a moderate life crisis, and more than 299 as a major life crisis. In terms of Selye's (1956) three stages of responding to stress, it could be said that the abusive parents had no sooner gone through the first phase of shock and countershock and had begun to enter the second stage of resistance when a new crisis came along, and they plunged into the third stage—exhaustion. It is this stage of exhaustion, when defenses are lowest and controls on acting out behavior are weakest, that abuse occurs.

An important question that remained for us, however, in understanding child abuse, was why a person who undergoes a life crisis would abuse a child as opposed to expressing the stress in some other way. If, as other investigators have found, excessive change can lead to illness, accident, injury, or emotional difficulties, why would it lead to violence toward a child in the case of some people? For child abuse to be an outcome of a life crisis, other factors must also be present.

The characteristics of the abusing parents must be considered a causal factor. Most abusive parents are products of what Helfer (1974) calls the "World of Abnormal Rearing." The cycle begins with parents having unrealistic expectations of their child. They expect to *receive* nuturing from their offspring, not give it. The child complies as best he or she can but, in the process, does not learn to trust. As a result, the child develops a sense of distrust, becomes isolated, and, consequently, has impaired social skills. When grown, this person is likely to pick for a mate someone with similar problems. Both parents marry with the expectations that their mate will nurture them and give them the kind of love they never received as children. Both are disappointed but one "gives in" and assumes the caretaker role most of the time. That person, the "loser" in the struggle for nurturing, decides to have a child, with the idea in mind that a baby will give the much-needed and never-received love. When the child fails to deliver on such a heavy demand, and the parent is under stress, abuse occurs, as violence is used in an effort to force the child into being a caretaker.

The child in the abusing family must also be considered as a contributing factor. The parent's abuse is directed at a "special" child, the one the parent perceives as being most in need of attention or care or the most threatening competitor to the parent seeking the same thing. At high risk of being physically abused are children who are premature, twins, retarded or handicapped, adopted, congenitally malformed, conceived during a mother's depressive illness, or children of mothers with frequent pregnancies. Sometimes the "specialness" is more imagined than real. The child may be singled out because he or she resembles some disliked relative or reminds the parents of something they dislike about themselves.

The final factor in our Psychosocial Stress Model is what we call "cultural scripts." By "cultural scripts" we mean the accepted and expected patterns of interaction between individuals in a society. One cultural script is embodied in the saying "Spare the rod and spoil the child," which reflects the attitude that violence towards children is not only acceptable but even necessary. Other cultural myths are those we call the "Madonna mother" myth and the "Gerber baby" myth. Both myths are perpetuated by the media, which portray all mothers as kind, loving, serene, organized "Supermoms" and all babies as cute, cuddly, clean, and easy to care for. When the facts do not match these idealized images, the potentially abusive parent experiences anger and/or guilt that further increases the family tension.

Treatment of Abusive Families

Using this Psychosocial Stress Model as a theoretical base in our approach to treating abusive parents, we concentrate on identifying and changing behaviors that contribute to the abuse. The first night parents enter our group (an ongoing group with new couples being added when space is available), we ask them to fill out a checklist of problems that are of possible concern to them (see Exhibit 1-1). We have found this to be a nonthreatening way for clients to identify and communicate to us the problems they are experiencing in their lives. Since the items on the checklist do not directly focus on the subject of child abuse, the parents feel safer in discussing the problems they mark.

Only occasionally does a parent turn in the checklist completely blank. When that happens, it is a useful diagnostic tool. The person who gives us a blank checklist, mumbling something to the effect that, ''I don't have any problems,'' is telling us that he or she is unwilling to give us *anything*. Our experience is that that is exactly what we end up with—nothing. We have learned over the years not to do battle with the parents by arguing that, indeed, they do have problems. We wouldn't win the argument anyway. Instead, we accept the blank checklist and make some comment like, ''It's a good thing you didn't check anything. We might have gotten confused. Now we know you're just here to help your spouse.'' This paradoxical technique gets us through a tense moment, but the fact remains that the parent who turns in a blank checklist is unlikely to come back to the group more than one or two times, and we are probably not going to effect a permanent change in the family. That has only happened once in the years we have been working with abusive parents. In that instance, the father turned in the blank sheet, came twice to therapy, and left town when his infant son died of the injuries the mother had inflicted and criminal charges for murder were filed against her.

Although the parents may be angry when they first come into the group, we make it clear that we played no role in their losing custody of the child or being forced to come to therapy. We describe our job as doing all we can to help the parents get their children back and that we can only do this if the situation in the family changes sufficiently for the

Exhibit 1-1

Problems Checklist

Name: _______________________

Date: _______________________

Which of the following are areas of concern to you?

(Check here)

__________ *Low self-image*—low opinion of self, think you're no good, can't do anything right.

__________ *Don't have friends*—keep to self a lot, isolated from others, feel alone.

__________ *Temper and/or impatience*—have a "short fuse," blow up easily, or get impatient with nearly everyone.

__________ *Dependent*—Depend heavily on spouse, can't make decisions yourself, can't make it without spouse or some other relative; often irresponsible.

__________ *Little support from spouse*—have to do most of decision-making yourself, can't depend on spouse to help with kids or to give "moral support," or to say nice things.

__________ *Stress*—feel under much pressure all the time from job, kids, house, finances or other reasons.

__________ *Child development and needs*—don't know much about the needs of babies and children at various ages and what to expect.

__________ *Sex*—little or no sexual satisfaction in marriage, frustration, arguments over sex.

__________ *Trust*—can't trust anyone, always being let down, look at people with suspicion.

__________ *Depression*—feel down and hopeless, have trouble getting things done and making decisions, life looks bleak.

__________ *Child is disappointment*—child isn't loving or doesn't do what you expect or seems different from other children.

__________ *Child care or management*—need to know much more about what to do for and with baby or child at various ages, and how to get child to "behave."

Make sure you have checked all the problems that are of concern to you.

Now look at the list of problems again and RANK them in terms of which are bigger problems and which are smaller problems.

For example, if temper/impatience is your biggest problem, put the number 1 by it in the list below. Then go down the list and see what is your second biggest problem. If trust is the second biggest, put a 2 by it.

Put numbers by all the problems that are of concern to you so you will rank them according to importance. If two are of EQUAL weight or importance, put the same number by each of the problems.

(Rank problems by putting number by each concern)

_________ Low self-image		_________ Child development and needs
_________ Don't have friends		_________ Sex
_________ Temper and/or impatience		_________ Trust
_________ Dependent		_________ Depression
_________ Little support from spouse		_________ Child is disappointment
_________ Stress		_________ Child care or management

child protective service workers to feel confident that the home is safe for the children to return. In cases where the parents have not lost custody of a child but insist that their only problem is that child welfare is in their lives, we point out that child welfare is not in *everyone's* life, and that we will help them figure out how to get free of that encumbrance. Our role, as we see it and explain it to the parents, is to make it possible for them to manage their children with less difficulty, so we can report back to the child protective workers that we think enough changes have been made so that the child can safely live with his or her parents. We are very direct in letting the parents know that if no changes are made, that is exactly what we will report. Since the parents sign treatment consent forms before they come to the group for the first meeting, they know we will be reporting on their progress to the caseworkers. A few parents opt to leave therapy rather than change. That is their right, of course, and those we worked with who took that option permanently lost custody of their children. Although those parents may indeed love their children as much as the parents who stick with therapy, they may simply feel incapable of parenting any longer, and we as therapists need to respect that decision.

The use of a group as a treatment modality helps to break down resistance even more rapidly. A new couple enters a group with seasoned members. Some of the parents have been in the group long enough to have their children returned, and all but the new couple have been attending long enough to see us as advocates instead of adversaries. If the new people express much resentment in their first group session or two, we will simply let the veteran members talk for a while about how they felt when they first came to the group. More often, this conversation goes on after the session when the couples stand around talking in the hall or go out together for coffee. The very fact that there are parents who have had a removed child returned is reassuring to the new couple. Because the group plays such an important role, we make it a point not to have more than one couple enter the group in any one week. Our experience is that after three or four weeks the parents' resentment at having been ordered to come to the group dissipates.

Because of the fine line between Rescuer and Persecutor (Karpman, 1968) in working with "coerced" clients, we think it is not possible to be both the caseworker and therapist to the same parents. In situations in which therapy with abusive parents is done by the child protection workers, it is essential that the therapist be a different worker than the caseworker who is handling the case. It is virtually impossible not to be seen as a persecutor by the parents when one holds the power to decide whether or not the parents' child is to be removed or returned. Even if there are only two workers in a unit, it is preferable for the workers to trade off with each other, so that neither is trying to be both psychotherapist and caseworker to the same parents.

Using the filled-in checklist, we begin working with the parents on the problems they say are of concern to them, even if those problems do not on the surface appear to be related to problems in dealing with their children. Once they feel safe with us, the parents will begin talking about their children. The most common problems we address with the parents are these: (1) symbiotic relationship; (2) isolation; (3) talking and sharing with mate; (4) impatience and/or temper; (5) child development and management; and (6) unemployment. Although not every couple has problems in all these areas, most of the couples do. A Goal Attainment Follow-Up Guide, as developed by Kiresuk and Sherman (1968), is constructed for each person in the group, setting 3-month goals for each area of concern. The guide is used both to record contracts between the therapists and clients and to measure change. Goal attainment scaling allows for more problems to be added as they are uncovered. For instance, depression was a problem we listed and worked on directly with some of the parents. With others, who were more mildly depressed, we found that as gains were made in breaking up the isolation and the symbiotic relationship, signs of the depression went away. Similarly, a problem of low self-image would be alleviated when there was improvement in the marriage. The formula for computing a goal attainment score enables us to assign weights of relative importance to each particular problem and then to arrive at a specific change score. Caseworkers for the parents have found the concreteness very helpful when reporting progress to the courts.

Symbiosis

Since we consider the symbiotic relationship central to abusive behavior, that problem area is usually given more weight than the other areas of concern. In the abusing family, as we have noted, there is a constant struggle to be in the "cared for" position. Symbiosis, as defined in transactional analysis terms by the Schiffs (1971) involves a competition to claim the Child role. The spouses struggle with each other over who is going to take care of whom, both physically and emotionally. In therapy, our goal is to break up the symbiosis by chipping away at the behaviors that reinforce it.

The difference between meeting one's needs through symbiosis and through autonomy is that the autonomous person is aware of his or her needs and consciously takes steps to meet them. In symbiosis, the person manipulates others into meeting his or her needs without considering whether they are willing or able to do so. The demand takes the form of passivity. Passivity, in the context of symbiosis means devoting one's energies to reestablishing a symbiotic relationship—as opposed to taking direct action to meet one's own needs. According to the Schiffs, there are four types of passive behavior: (1) doing nothing, (2) overadaptation, (3) agitation, and (4) incapacitation or violence. The person who does nothing mobilizes all his or her energy to avoid responding when confronted with a problem. Doing nothing is usually accompanied by not thinking. The person who overadapts tries to solve a problem according to someone else's expectations rather than deciding on his or her own solution and carrying it out. Again, the element of not thinking is involved. Agitation is nongoal-directed activity, such as wiggling one's foot or chain smoking, which may relieve tension to an extent but does nothing to solve the problem. Although violence and incapacitation seem to be opposites, they both serve to discharge the energy built up by passivity and they both force someone else to take over, be that "someone" the police or hospital personnel.

In group therapy, we work on teaching spouses how not to be forced into taking responsibility for the other one and how to be more responsible in getting one's needs met individually. For example, one parent is typically handling all the discipline in the family, therein assuming the Parent role. That person is also the one who is likely to have abused the child or children in the family. We would make a contract with that parent to leave all physical discipline, such as spankings, to the other parent. Such a contract is readily agreed to by the parent carrying all the responsibility, while the passive partner may put up some resistance. The contract serves to highlight the imbalance in parenting in the family and gives both parents an opportunity to negotiate about child care.

The indicators of symbiosis are often quite obvious: a wife who answers each time her husband is asked a question; a husband who makes all the spending decisions because his wife "goes crazy" with the checkbook; a husband whose "back goes out" every time his wife asks him to keep the kids while she visits her relatives. In the group, we take examples of the symbiosis as they appear, ask if that arrangement is a problem (it always is to at least one partner), and negotiate a contract for change.

Social Isolation

Social isolation is a second major problem we see in abusive families. The isolated parent has never learned to reach out for help in times of crisis, and often there is no one outside the family for support. This isolation is even more critical for young parents who have moved to an urban area geographically removed from anyone they know. In a study in Los Angeles (Lenoski, 1973) comparing 674 abusing parents with a control group of 500 nonabusers, it was reported that 80.9% of the abusing parents said they preferred to resolve crises alone, compared with 43.3% of the controls; 43.3% of the abusing parents preferred to be alone, compared with 20% of the controls. Only 10.5% of the abusing parents had listed telephone numbers, compared with 88% of the controls. Abusive parents are often lonely people. They are cut off from others both in fact and feeling. They have few contacts with people outside their immediate families, if at all. So our work in this area focuses on ways to break the isolation and start successful contacts with others.

Being in a group is an important first step. Once a week, for an hour and a half, the parents are with people they have something in common with and with whom they can discuss personal problems without being criticized or blamed. Friendships, although sometimes awkward, are formed. Members of the group visit each other from time to time. Problems that arise in the new friendships are discussed in the group. Telephone numbers are exchanged, including ours. We make it a point to let the group members know that we are available by giving them both our office and home numbers. (We also make it clear that we take good care of ourselves by telling them that if they are going to have a crisis and want us involved to have the crisis after 7:00 A.M. and before 10:30 P.M. They must get the message since we have had calls from the parents only during those hours.) Gradually, the parents learn to reach out in times of crisis. They also learn that social support helps alleviate stress in their lives. Behavior modification contracts are used to further break down isolation. Parents contract to meet their neighbors, to get listed telephone numbers, and, for housebound wives, to get jobs where they can be around people and make friends.

Talking and Sharing with Mate

Marital problems are uniformly present for couples entering the group. The most common complaints are ''We don't communicate'' or ''He/she never talks/listens to me.'' Initially, many of the couples deny they have any problems with their marriages, but by the end of the first few group sessions, the problems and hostilities surface.

Our approach is to take the marital complaints as they come up and negotiate behavioral contracts that both of the partners agree to. One woman in the group, for instance, complained that her husband would never talk to her when he got home from work. Instead, he would turn on three television sets—one for each of the major channels—and read the papers or go outside to mow the lawn (twice a week) as soon as the news ended. She lamented about not being able to get her husband's attention except in a crisis—like the day she fractured her baby boy's arm. The husband, in turn, was unhappy about his wife's never wanting to visit with his relatives. The two contracted that when the husband first came home, he would spend a minimum of 15 minutes just visiting with his wife and letting her talk to him. In turn, his wife agreed to socialize with his relatives once a month. Striking bargains like this is not uncommon in the group, and the couple usually stick to the agreements since they are made in front of other people and each partner has something to gain. It makes no difference how insignificant the change is as long as there is some change in the direction of improving the marital relationship.

Child Development and Management

Most of the parents enter our group badly informed about children's needs and how to manage them without physical discipline. Soon after entering the group, each couple is given a chart describing the developmental stages of children and the corresponding needs. The chart presents in a simple way what a child needs at various ages and stages and lists the do's and don't's for the parents at each stage. Parents contract to learn those parts of the chart that apply to their own children and to report back to the group about their efforts at practicing the do's and don't's.

One couple did not know what to do about their 4-year-old's insistence that there were monsters in his room. Bedtime had become a nightly battle, with the little boy being sent to bed each night with a swat from his father's belt. After being reassured that many children that age believe in monsters, they came up with a clever way of reassuring the boy that it was safe to go into his room at night. The father brought out a can of "monster spray" (room deodorant) and sprayed under the boy's bed each night. The procedure worked well enough to let everyone go to sleep without a family uproar.

At each group session, we do a problem-solving exercise on child management, using examples from a book by Smith and Smith (1966). We hand out copies of chapters on specific issues, such as setting and enforcing rules. After discussing the content, we go around the group asking each member to take one of the problems presented and choose one of the multiple-choice answers to it. Many questions are generated from these exercises, and it gives us an opportunity to see what deficiencies the parents have in their information about parenting. We maintain a lending library for parents to borrow books on child management and introductory material on transactional analysis. Depending on the parent's reading ability and interest in reading, we assign books that are mostly pictures on up to more sophisticated material, such as Gordon's *Parent*

Effectiveness Training (1970). In between are books like *Children: The Challenge* (Dreikurs, 1964) and *Dare to Discipline* (Dobson, 1970). Parents contract to read the books and discuss sections from them.

Role playing is an additional technique we use in teaching child management. If a couple is having a particular problem with their child, we might ask a group member to play the role of the child, acting out the objectional behavior. One of the parents then demonstrates how he or she is attempting to correct the child. The group's feedback on the interaction is invaluable. When one young mother was showing how she attempted to get her 2-year-old (being played by a woman in the group) to stop playing with a dangerous object, the mother immediately started fussing and fighting with the child. The idea of distracting the baby with something more interesting had not even occurred to her until the members of the group suggested it.

Temper and/or Impatience

The temper levels of people in our group range to both ends of the spectrum. A number of "acting-out" parents describe themselves as "hot-tempered" or having a "short fuse." The more passive partners frequently have trouble expressing anger at all. For this latter group, we often find it necessary to teach assertiveness training to help them get their needs met.

For all the group, we schedule a weekly relaxation exercise. The last 15 minutes of each session, we play a relaxation tape that uses breathing techniques and visual imagery. Occasionally, we substitute a progressive relaxation exercise. In addition to this weekly group exercise, some parents contract to do 5-minute segments of breathing and imagery a certain number of times during the week between meetings. Since we began incorporating the relaxation tape as a regular feature of the group session, we have found that the members change faster and settle into the group more quickly. The parents report that the relaxation training is particularly useful when they start feeling uptight at home or work or feel they are about to have an outburst of temper.

Employment

A number of parents in our group have some kind of employment stress which existed at the time they abused their children. For some, the stress is from being laid off from work, for others it is the result of working two jobs or double shifts, and for still others, the stress is from being dissatisfied with the jobs they have. Our role here is to provide information about job training, job banks, and stress management on the job. The latter includes teaching individuals how to handle their upsets when they don't like what happens at work. Sometimes the group members exchange information on where jobs can be found, and, at one point, several members ended up working at the same place, where they could share rides going and coming.

Some of the women in the group are teen-agers who never worked before their babies were born and who spend their days watching soap operas after their children are taken away. They are lonely and yet afraid to risk taking on a job. We use contracts initially just to get them to apply for work. Once they do start working, they make friends and the isolation, as well as their dependence on their mates, starts to break up.

Managing Stress

Stress is not only the central problem for most parents in the employment area, it is also an element in each of the other five problems. Therefore, another intervention we make consists of providing stress management techniques. Many of the parents customarily deal with stressors either by counterattacking (blowing up, becoming aggressive) or by withdrawal (retreating from the problem). We spend considerable time teaching how to confront in an assertive but not aggressive way.

A second coping behavior these parents lack is cognitive appraisal skills. Most of the parents, when they enter therapy, do not recognize that the intensity of the stress they experience is determined by how they evaluate or interpret the problem before them. When they are given rational emotive techniques for managing their internal dialogues, they have another method to keep themselves from getting distressed when the job of child rearing seems overwhelming.

An additional coping method we emphasize is doing something about the physical effects of stress. Many parents contract to run or exercise daily, which helps them greatly in relieving tension. The relaxation exercises also provide relief.

Conclusions on Coercive Therapy

It is certainly preferable to work with clients who seek therapy, are cooperative, and willing to change. Unfortunately, as therapists dealing with the life-threatening problem of child abuse, we do not always have the luxury of waiting for our clients to become motivated and enter therapy on their own. Our primary goal in working with abusive parents is to make the home safe for the children in it. Unless their parents undergo treatment, the children remain at risk.

While the parents may not want to be in therapy, they do want their lives to work better, and they want to be able to cope with their children more successfully. When parents are "forced" into therapy, the odds are greatly enhanced that they will indeed learn more effective coping skills. All the parents who come to our group are, by their presence, making an affirmative statement of their willingness to do something about their troubled lives. The words they say are not nearly as significant as the message they are conveying by coming to therapy week after week. We choose to interpret their being present as a desire to proceed with treatment.

Our results seem to support our interpretation. Most of the parents do improve their parenting skills to the point that their children are returned and safely allowed to remain at home. Even more important, they stop expecting their children to take care of them and instead they begin to become the caretakers. The parents learn to fulfill their emotional needs in more constructive ways than by turning to their children. Our experience with these parents bears out the behavior therapy principles that if people will practice a new behavior by going to therapy and doing homework assignments, their feelings as well as their actions will change.

REFERENCES

Burns, D.D. *Feeling good: The new mood therapy.* New York: Morrow, 1980.

Dobson, J. *Dare to discipline.* Wheaton, Ill.: Tyndale House, 1970.

Dreikurs, R. *Children: The challenge.* New York: Hawthorn, 1964.

Gelles, R.J. Child abuse as psychopathology: A sociological critique and reformulation. *American Journal of Orthopsychiatry*, 1973, *43*, 611–621.

Gil, D.G. Physical abuse of children: Findings and implications of a nationwide survey. *Pediatrics*, 1969, *44*, 862.

Gil, D.G. *Violence against children.* Cambridge, Mass.: Harvard University Press, 1970.

Gordon, T. *Parent effectiveness training.* New York: Peter H. Wyden, 1970.

Helfer, R.E. *A self-instructional program on child abuse and neglect.* Committee on Infant and Preschool Child, American Academy of Pediatrics, Chicago, Ill., and National Center for the Prevention and Treatment of Child Abuse and Neglect, Denver, Colo., 1974.

Holmes, T.H., & Rahe, R.H. The social readjustment rating scale. *Journal of Psychosomatic Research*, 1967, *11*, 213–218.

Justice, B., & Justice, R. *The abusing family.* New York: Human Sciences Press, 1976.

Justice, B., & Justice, R. *The broken taboo: Sex in the family.* New York: Human Sciences Press, 1979.

Karpman, S.B. Fairy tales and script drama analysis. *Transactional Analysis Bulletin,* 1968, 7(26).

Kempe, C.H. Paediatric implications of the battered baby syndrome. *Archives of Disease in Childhood,* 1971, *46* (28), 28–37.

Kempe, C.H., & Helfer, R.E. (Eds.). *Helping the battered child and his family.* Philadelphia: Lippincott, 1972.

Kiresuk, T.J., & Sherman, R.E. Goal attainment scaling: A general method for evaluating comprehensive community mental health programs. *Community Mental Health Journal,* 1968, *4,* 443–453.

Lenoski, E.F. Translating injury data into preventive services: Physical child abuse. Unpublished paper, University of Southern California Medical Center, Division of Emergency Medicine, Los Angeles, 1973.

Maletzky, B.M. Self-referred versus court-referred sexually deviant patients: Success with assisted covert sensitization. *Behavior Therapy,* 1980, *11,* 306–314.

Schiff, A.W. & Schiff, J. Passivity. *Transactional Analysis Journal,* 1971, *1,* 1.

Selye, H. *The stress of life.* New York: McGraw-Hill, 1956.

Smith, J.M., & Smith, D.E.P. *Child management: A program for parents.* Ann Arbor, Mich.: Ann Arbor Publishers, 1966.

Straus, M., Gelles, R.J., & Steinmetz, S.K. *Behind closed doors: Violence in the American family.* New York: Doubleday/Anchor, 1979.

2. The Epidemiology of Violence in a CMHC Setting: A Violence Epidemic?

Laurence R. Barnhill, Ph.D.
Coordinator
Outpatient and Emergency Services
South Central Community Mental Health Center
Bloomington, Indiana

Margaret F. Squires, Ph.D.
Addictions Therapist
South Central Community Mental Health Center
Bloomington, Indiana

Gordon Gibson, M.S.
Director of Evaluation Research
South Central Community Mental Health Center
Bloomington, Indiana

Two

MUCH RECENT COMMENTARY FROM MENTAL HEALTH professionals and activist client advocates has suggested that the mental health field has generally avoided addressing the issue of interpersonal, and, more specifically, intrafamilial violence (O'Brien, 1971; Martin, 1976). Newly formed professional and lay groups focusing on issues of child abuse and spouse abuse have noted the apparent epidemic proportions of these problems in the United States (Helfer & Kempe, 1972; Gelles, 1972; Gil, 1970; Straus, Gelles, & Steinmetz, 1980). The large number of new programs for treating these difficulties in communities across the country demonstrates an increased awareness that mental health services have some responsibility for assisting individuals, families, and communities with the problem of violence (APA, 1974).

While there have been some recent major attempts to study the epidemiology of violence in the country at large (Straus, Gelles, & Steinmetz, 1980), probably the most relevant issue for mental health professionals is determining the extent of violence in a clinical population. The first attempt to determine the extent of violence in an agency–client population found that more than 7% of a Detroit Family Service Agency's cases involved violence (Ball, 1977). There have been no comparable data for community mental health center (CMHC) populations.

The goal of this study was to determine the incidence and general characteristics of violence among clients of a midwestern small-town CMHC. How many clients have such a problem and how serious is the problem? What is the nature of the relationships in which violence occurs? Answers to these questions could indicate whether or not a ''violence epidemic'' exists. These data could also suggest the need for specialized treatment programs for this population. In addition, such information could help identify needs for staff training in the multidisciplinary field of violence and its control.

Methodology

Setting

Our study was conducted in a midwestern four-county area with a total population of 200,000. There are marked variations among the counties with regard to socioeconomic class status (rural poverty to average family incomes), age and population density (the sparsely populated areas have higher proportions of elderly people), life styles (rural agrarian, small industry, and university community), and availability of human services (few in some areas, many in others). Community mental health outpatient clinics are located in each of the four counties. Inpatient facilities are located only in the largest and most central county.

Measure

The data were collected using the Violence Needs Assessment, an instrument based on Ball's previous study (1977) modified for our purposes. (See Exhibit 2-1.) The form is primarily descriptive, gathering data on the characteristics of persons involved in violence, the types and severity of the violence, where and when the case was identified, and the relationships involved in the violence. Much of these data are straightforward, the only innovation being a rating scale of the level of violence. The definition of violence used for the ratings was intended to be concrete and specific, yet also to provide a general statement. (See Gelles, 1972, for a discussion of definition problems.)

Procedure

Data were collected on all routine and emergency admissions and all discharges in the four-county area for a 3-month period in the winter of 1978-1979. The assessment was completed by the intake worker or therapist with responsibility for the case. In order to decrease data loss, the assessment was completed for all cases rather than just those identified as involving violence. Data for clients who were both admitted and discharged during the study period were tabulated only once, at discharges, in order to eliminate redundancies.

Exhibit 2-1 Violence Needs Assessment

Client Name: _________________ Date of Intake: ___________ Case Number: _____

CMHC Staff Name: _____________________ Date of this Report: ______________

I. Concern is expressed *(Check all that apply)*:

( ) At intake   ( ) No evidence of, nor concern
( ) During treatment   about, violence (skip rest of form)

II. Concern is expressed by *(Check only one)*:
( ) Victim or intended victim
( ) Assaulter or potential assaulter
( ) Both victim and assaulter
( ) Other (Specify, e.g., family, police, therapist, etc.): _____________

III. Characteristics of Victim and Assaulter *(Check as applies)*:

A. Victim or intended victim: ___ Age ( ) Male   ( ) Adult
                                            ( ) Female   ( ) Child

B. Assaulter or potential assaulter: ___ Age ( ) Male   ( ) Adult
                                            ( ) Female   ( ) Child

C. Relationship of victim and assaulter: ( ) Marital Relationship
                                             ( ) Parent-Child Relationship
                                             ( ) Other (Specify): _________

IV. Level of Violence for the Current Incident *(Use the scaling below to rate the level of violence from 0 to 5)*:
Current Level: ____________

V. Level of Violence for Past Incidents *(Use the scaling below to rate the level of violence from 0 to 5)*:
Past Level: ______________

0   None, or socially sanctioned, e.g., spanking

1   Rare hitting (slapping), usually only one way, and when under stress. Repetitive shouting matches, verbal threats not carried out. Property damage, thefts. Reported hostile-aggressive impulses, not carried out.

2   Repetitive hitting, and/or grabbing, throwing objects, serious threat, major attack on property.

3   Extreme fighting without weapon, attempt to hurt, or threat with weapon, but not in direct attack.

4   Attempt to injure with weapon or other.

5   Attempt to kill or seriously injure.

Definition of "violence": An act (or attempt or threat) of harming another that is physically destructive. That is, pushing, slapping, punching, kicking, knifing, shooting, hitting with an object, or throwing an object with the intent of inflicting bodily harm.

Table 2-1 Classification of Clinical Caseload by Client Report of Concern about Violence

	Number	*Percent*
Current Concern	205	24.5
Past Concern Only	126	15.0
No Concern Reported	506	60.5
Total	837	100.0

FINDINGS

Results were grouped into three major areas, beginning with a census of current and past violence identified at various points in the service delivery system. The second area is the seriousness of the violence, including data on both the intensity or "level" of violence and the number of violent relationships involved in the case. In the third major area, data are presented on the age and gender of the victims and assailants and their relationships to each other.

Identification of Violence Cases

Table 2-1 displays the total number of cases, 837, involved in the study. Of these, 39.5%, or 331 individuals, reported a concern about violence. This total is in striking contrast to Ball's (1977) earlier report of 7% (of over 1,500 cases) as violent. Violence was a *current* concern in 24.5%, or 205 cases, and was a concern in the *past only* for an additional 15.0%, or 126 cases. Since this area of the country is not particularly characterized by a high degree of violence, the fact that a current concern about a problem of violence was expressed in one-fourth of the cases appears to be strong evidence that the problem warrants serious concern.

Table 2-2 presents data on the type of service being utilized as well as when the case was identified (admission or discharge). Inpatient cases are all listed as discharges since treatment is short term (up to 2 weeks) and admissions and discharges would include essentially the same cases. Cases that included use of both outpatient and inpatient services were classified as "inpatients." Almost half (49.4%) of the 77 inpatients reported some difficulty with violence. Although much of this violence was within the family (see Table 2-6 below), the inpatient group also included numerous examples of violence toward caretakers (inpatient staff, emergency personnel, etc.).

Table 2-2 Client Concern about Violence by Type of Mental Health Service Being Utilized

	Inpatient Discharges	Outpatient Admissions	Outpatient Discharges
Number of Clients	77	430	330
Violence Reported (%)	49.4	48.4	25.8
No Violence Reported (%)	50.6	51.6	74.2

The outpatient population of 430 admissions and 330 discharges included 38.6%, or 293 patients, with a past or present concern about violence. Outpatient admissions are similar to inpatient cases, with 48.4% of the patients reporting a violence concern.

One factor contributing to the more frequent identification of incidents of violence in new cases (admissions) may have been the new CMHC programs on child abuse and spouse abuse, which led to increased referrals for this type of problem. Since the programs were quite small at the time of the study, however, other factors must also have contributed to the marked discrepancy in numbers of cases identified on admission and at discharge. One of the most likely is a Hawthorne effect (Homans, 1958), whereby the process of measurement increased staff members' awareness of the potential for such problems.

Seriousness of the Violence

Table 2-3 presents data on the 287 violence cases for which we have complete ratings of the level of violence. Of the 173 cases with a *current* violence concern, a smooth positively skewed curve can be inferred. Almost half of the cases are in the lowest category, level one, of rare violence, threats, or reported impulses. Approximately one-fourth are at level 2, including repetitive minor violence, serious threats, or serious attacks on property (for example, arson). Thus, as might be expected, the majority of violence occurs at less serious levels. Eleven percent of the violence cases, however, included categories 4 and 5, attempts to seriously injure, maim, or kill.

In *past only* concerns about violence, the same smooth curve is not obtained, though the general trend is similar. That is, most of the violence again occurred at the lowest two levels, and the least at the highest levels. Since raters were instructed to rate the highest level of violence

Table 2-3 Percentage of Cases of Violence by Level of Violence and Type of Concern

Level of Violence	Current Concern, 173 Cases	Past Concern Only, 114 Cases
1. Rare Hitting, Verbal	49.1	33.4
2. Repetitive Hitting	26.6	36.0
3. Extreme Fighting	13.3	18.4
4. Attempted Injury (weapon)	8.7	6.1
5. Attempted Murder, Maiming	2.3	6.1
Total	100.0	100.0

reported, it seems reasonable to expect a trend toward somewhat higher ratings when all of the past was considered.

We feel it is important to note that while we define levels 1 and 2 as "lower" levels, we do not define them as not serious. Level 1 violence of, for example, an occasional slug or a threat such as "you say (or do) that again and I'll smash your face" should not be defined away as "not serious" violence. It is objectively serious in that previous violence is the best predictor of future (at times more extreme) violence, and it can be subjectively serious to a potential victim who may live in fear (Barnhill, 1980a).

Table 2-4 addresses another dimension related to seriousness of violence: the number of violent relationships in which a client reported involvement. Of the 331 violent cases, 69.8% (231 cases) reported violence in one relationship; 30.2% (100 cases) reported multiple violent relationships. Again we find a relatively smooth, though steeper, positively skewed curve, with the majority of cases reporting the fewest violent relationships and a few cases reporting many.

Gender, Age, and Relationships Involved in Violence

Table 2-5 presents the gender breakdown of assaulters and victims. Four-fifths (79.6%) of the assaulters were male, whereas one-fifth were female. Victims were nearly the reverse, with females being the victim in 67.2% of the cases and males in 29.5% of the cases.

Gender interactions can be compared by examining the relationships involved in the violent incidents. In the majority (57.4%) of the cases, the assaulter is male and the victim is female. The next most common gender interaction (22.2%) involves male assaulters and male victims.

Table 2-4 Comparison of Cases of Violence by the Number of Violent Relationships

Reported Violent Relationships	Number	Percent	Cumulative Percent
One Relationship	231	69.8	69.8
Two Relationships	59	17.8	87.6
Three Relationships	25	7.6	95.2
Four Relationships	8	2.4	97.6
Five or More Relationships	8	2.4	100.0
Total	331	100.0	

Thus, in this population, men are much more likely to be assaultive, and to assault women more than they assault other men. Women, on the other hand, while assaultive more rarely, attack male or female victims in roughly equal numbers.

In order to determine who is seeking help, data were gathered on a subsample of 146 cases regarding the role of the client in the violent situation. In these cases, the assailant was the client in the majority of cases (52.1%), and the victim was in treatment in 32.9% of the cases. Both were clients in 8.2% of the cases. The client was a witness or otherwise indirectly involved in 6.8% of the cases. It is noteworthy that in over 60% of the cases, the assaulter was in treatment. This is in contrast to reports by some (e.g., Martin, 1976) that the "victim is blamed" while the assaulter escapes scrutiny. It is also of pragmatic interest that such a significant number of clients are identifying a problem in aggression and seeking treatment.

Data regarding ages of victims and assaulters revealed a substantial child abuse population. While only 6.6% of assaulters were under 18 years of age, 29.1% of the victims were under 18. Victims' ages ranged from under 1 year to 67 years, with a mean of 24.3 years and a mode of

Table 2-5 Percentage of Incidents of Violence by Gender Interaction with the Roles of Assaulter and Victim

	Gender of Victim	
Gender of Assaulters	Female	Male
Females	9.8%	10.6%
Males	54.4%	22.2%

Note: There were 397 incidents of violence for this crosstabulation.

Table 2-6 Cases of Violence by the Type of Relationship of the Client Involved in the Incident

Type of Relationship	Number	Percent	Cumulative Percent
Spouse	153	32.4	32.4
Parent-Child	175	37.1	69.5
Sibling	15	3.2	72.7
Extended Family	13	2.8	75.5
Known Nonfamily	80	16.9	92.4
Strangers	36	7.6	100.0
Total	472	100.0	

25 years. Assaulters represented a somewhat narrower range, from 6 to 64 years, with a mean and mode of 30 years.

Table 2-6 combines data on all violent relationships (not just one count per case), categorized by the nature of the relationship(s) involved in the violence. We have completed relationship data on 472 incidents of violence in the 331 cases. Spouse abuse and child abuse are roughly equivalent, and when combined account for more than two-thirds of all cases of violence reported. Adding the small percentage of sibling violence yields 72.7% of all incidents as occurring within the nuclear family. An additional 2.8% of the incidents occurred in the extended families. Thus, 75.5% of all incidents were family related. Known nonfamily includes most of the rest of the cases (16.9%). This category includes cohabitants, perceived rivals, coworkers, neighbors, etc. Strangers or unknown account for only 7.6% of violent incidents. These latter were primarily barroom fights, or assaults on caretakers, though one individual (inpatient) reported he had been assaulted by a Martian (he had clearly been assaulted by someone).

DISCUSSION

Clearly the major conclusion of this study is that violence is far more frequent among CMHC clientele than expected. Whereas previous Family Service Agency data indicated that 7% of its caseload had such a problem, these data demonstrate that 39.5% of these CMHC cases have or have had a concern about violence. This concern appears more common in inpatient cases (49.4%) than outpatient cases (38.6%), yet the frequency is high in both contexts.

This level of reporting has surprised even those of us committed to studying violence as an important, if little recognized, clinical problem. It seems remarkable that this amount of violence has escaped professional commentary and measurement until recently. Webster's definition of "epidemic" initially includes "widespread occurrence " and secondarily "said especially of a contagious disease" (1956). The present study and other evidence (Steinmetz, 1977; Straus, Gelles, & Steinmetz, 1980) indicates that intrafamilial violence is widespread and may be transmitted between family members (Eron, Walden, & Lefkowitz, 1971; Steinmetz, 1977). It appears clearly to be of epidemic proportion.

The striking discrepancy between the number of violence cases reported in new outpatient admissions and those found in outpatient discharge data on previous clients also deserves comment. It seems apparent that the process of measurement had a significant impact on the perceptions of the staff involved; new outpatient cases were seen to be almost twice as likely to have a violence concern as cases being terminated (48.4% rather than 25.8%).

With regard to the question of seriousness of the violence, the two measures of level and number of violent relationships showed a similar pattern. Most of the violence cases were of the lowest level of violence and, similarly, most cases reported only one violent relationship. Fewer cases reported a higher level of violence or multiple violent relationships. It is important, however, to note again that even low-level violence and single episodes can have serious consequences and thus should not necessarily be defined as "not serious."

The categories of age and gender involvement in violence provided evidence that, in this population, men are much more likely to be violent than women; they are also more likely to pick female targets. Adults are more violent than children, according to these results, and are somewhat disproportionately likely to choose a victim under 18. It is also noteworthy that both victims and assaulters are well represented in the client pool; the perpetrators of violence *are* seeking treatment.

In a finding that provides confirmation of earlier work, approximately 75% of the violence cases were intrafamilial. Violence towards spouses and children predominated, each one accounting for roughly one-third of the violence cases. This high degree of violence in families certainly suggests some familial transmission of the problem, including learning, heredity, or both. These data also suggest that intervention programs for violence should involve a family perspective, if not actually utilizing family therapy (Barnhill, 1980b).

Since so many of the findings of this study are new and not replicated (e.g., amount and level of violence, gender interaction, the Hawthorne effect on reporting), it is hoped that future research will address some of these issues. Expanding the data base to include all or most social service, health care, and legal agencies in a given community would be a valuable step. Such data would provide some perspective on violence cases in clinical populations as well as move toward a communitywide analysis of all violence cases reported to community agencies. Another important step would be to compare the incidence of violence in a clinical sample and a "normal" sample of the same population. In terms of clinical treatment of these cases, a critically important area would be longitudinal studies of the course of violent behavior over time. Closely related would be studies of treatment effectiveness, focusing on both immediate and long-term results.

In summary, it appears that community clinics and family-oriented therapists may play a key role in efforts to deal with violence. Both assaulters and victims come for treatment, and in much larger numbers than previously acknowledged. This "epidemic" suggests the need for specialized clinical programs and also the mandate to work with other community case finders and resource providers in order to address the needs of the individuals, families, and communities involved (Barnhill, Bloomgarden, Berghorn, Squires & Siracusa, 1980).

REFERENCES

American Psychiatric Association. *Clinical aspects of the violent individual.* Task Force Report 8. Washington, D.C.: APA, 1974.

Ball, M. Issues of violence in family casework. *Social Casework,* 1977, *58,* 3–12.

Barnhill, L. Clinical assessment of intrafamilial violence. *Hospital and Community Psychiatry,* 1980, *31,* 543–547.(a)

Barnhill, L. Basic interventions for violence in families. *Hospital and Community Psychiatry,* 1980, *31,* 547–551.(b)

Barnhill, L., Bloomgarden, R., Berghorn, G., Squires, M., & Siracusa, A. Clinical and community interventions in violence in families. In L. Wolberg & M. Aronson (Eds.), *Group and family therapy–1980.* New York: Stratton Medical Book Corp., 1980.

Eron, L., Walden, L., & Lefkowitz, M. *Learning aggression in children.* New York: Pergamon, 1971.

Gelles, R. *The violent home.* Beverly Hills, Calif.: Sage, 1972.

Gil, D. *Violence against children: Physical child abuse in the United States.* Cambridge, Mass.: Harvard University Press, 1970.

Helfer, R., & Kempe, C. *Helping the battered child and his family.* Philadelphia: Lippincott, 1972.

Homans, F. Group factors in worker productivity. In E. Maccoby, T. Newcombe, & E. Hartley (Eds.), *Readings in social psychology* (3rd ed.). New York: Holt, Rinehart, & Winston, 1958.

Martin, D. *Battered wives.* New York: Pocket Books, 1976.

O'Brien, J. Violence in divorce prone families. *Journal of Marriage and the Family,* 1971, *33,* 692–698.

Steinmetz, S. *Cycle of violence.* New York: Praeger, 1977.

Straus, M., Gelles, R., & Steinmetz, S. *Behind closed doors: Violence in the American family.* New York: Doubleday Anchor, 1980.

Webster's New World Dictionary. New York: World Publishing, 1956.

3. Biological Contributions to Family Violence

Frank A. Elliott, M.D.
Emeritus Professor, Neurology
University of Pennsylvania Medical School
Philadelphia, Pennsylvania
Consultant
Pennsylvania Hospital
Philadelphia, Pennsylvania

Three

SINCE THE BRAIN IS THE ORGAN OF THOUGHT, EMOTION, AND behavior, to discuss intrafamilial violence solely in terms of family dynamics and environmental stress is like considering a car's performance without reference to the efficiency of its engine. Yet for many years most sociological studies of the subject have paid little more than lip service to biological factors such as genetics, hormonal disorders, developmental defects, and acquired damage, which affect literally millions in the United States and which necessarily impair the adaptive potential of many. Gross neurological disorders such as mental retardation, cerebral palsy, and brain damage from trauma or encephalitis are recognized and allowed for, but more subtle biological contributions to behavioral disorders are apt to pass unnoticed. For instance, Horowitz (1982) found evidence of minimal brain dysfunction in 37% of 40 seriously disturbed individuals admitted to an adolescent treatment unit, yet the organic factor had been recognized by their psychiatrists in only five cases. In 286 personal cases of episodic violence, most of it directed at family members, brain defects were found in all but 18 cases (Elliott, in press). The prevalence of positive findings in this series was partly a result of selection bias in the type of case referred to a neurological department and partly due to the method of clinical examination and the use of the CT scan.

Insufficient attention has been paid to the work of many psychiatrists, psychologists, and neurophysiologists over the past 50 years on the role of neurological disorders in antisocial behavior. In 1936 Healy and Bronner reported that symptoms and signs of organic brain dysfunction were more common in child delinquents than in their nondelinquent siblings, and in 1942 Hill reported a high incidence of abnormal EEGs in aggressive adult psychopaths. In 1953 Thompson described abnormal neurological findings in the majority of a large group of psychopathic delinquents and criminals, and in 1970 Monroe reported a high prevalence of neurological soft signs, abnormal EEGs, and abnormal neuropsychological test results in both criminals and noncriminal psychiatric cases. Mark and Ervin (1970) published a small classic on the relationship between violence and brain damage, and in a landmark paper Bach-Y-Rita, Lion, Climent, and Ervin (1971) described a wide range of neuropathology in patients suffering from episodic dyscontrol; this has been confirmed by others. Neurological, radiological, and psychometric indications of organic disorders have also been found in borderline syndromes (Andrulonis, 1980) and atypical schizophrenias (Bellak, 1979). Many studies have reinforced Monroe's report (1970) of organic defects in antisocial personality disorders, including the classical psychopath (Mednick & Christiansen, 1977; Reid, 1978; Hare & Schalling, 1978; and Yeudall & Fromm-Rauch, 1979).

The use of the CT scan for the investigation of behavioral problems has shown much unsuspected pathology in cases of episodic dyscontrol (Elliott, 1978, in press) and in the schizophrenias. The cerebral atrophy found in many schizophrenics was demonstrated by old-fashioned encephalography about 50 years ago (Moore, 1933). There are indications that the Positron Emission Scanner and the Nuclear Magnetic Resonance Scan will uncover an even greater number of defects, including structural lesions and localized chemical and/or metabolic defects.

The emphasis given in this paper to the prevalence of developmental or acquired brain defects in relation to violent behavior is not intended to denigrate the role of psychodynamics or social stresses. It is hardly surprising that a flawed brain, like a flawed computer, is more likely to give wrong answers than a normal brain if the flaws are situated in sensitive areas such as the frontal or temporal lobes, or the limbic system, which is so intimately concerned with the expression and control of the emotions. Nevertheless, many brain-damaged individuals with serious physical handicaps escape social and emotional impairment.

HOW ORGANIC DISORDERS CAN CONTRIBUTE TO FAMILY STRIFE

One of the most disruptive and serious forms of antisocial behavior associated with organic neurological disorders is episodic dyscontrol, usually in the form of unpredictable attacks of uncontrollable rage in response to minor provocation (Mark & Ervin, 1970). Other forms are episodic sexual dyscontrol and episodic alcoholic binges. Even the anti-social activities of the "organic" psychopath tend to be episodic (Cleck-ley, 1976).

Other symptoms, though less dramatic, can be very trying (Anderson, 1972). Difficulty with thinking and a limited vocabulary hinders interper-sonal relationships and can lead to frustration and anger. The male, who usually has less verbal facility than the female, finds that when he is verbally assailed, it is easier to hit than to talk. Many brain-damaged individuals lack perception and miss the significance of the cues that are so essential to smooth social life—facial expression, tone of voice, and gestures—with the result that they often fail to perceive the frustration, anger, or grief of others. Some do not recognize their own anger and fail to understand why they alienate others; so they project blame. As a result of limited capacity for abstract thought they often fail to see the ultimate consequences of their impulsive and ill-considered actions. Some lack a normal sense of fear, which makes them accident prone; recurrent head injuries figure largely in the histories of many cases of minimal brain dysfunction. Other troublesome ingredients, which occur in varying com-binations, are hyperactivity or apathy, distractability, perseveration (e.g., persistence with a threadbare subject or argument), defective judgment, poor reasoning ability, lack of a capacity to fantasize, humorlessness, and specific learning problems (notably dyslexia, dysgraphia, dyscalculia, difficulty in spelling, and weakness of sequential memory). The brain-damaged are often unduly clumsy and maladroit, and untidy. They start programs and soon lose interest. Antisocial features include egocentricity, shallow or absent capacity for empathy with others, lack of social con-science, thievery, untruthfulness, tactlessness, callous brutality, fire set-ting, a tendency to gravitate into bad company, and a special liability to substance abuse. They usually have a low tolerance for psychological stress and are prone to catastrophic reactions.

The effect of these and other symptoms of brain damage on family life is eloquently described by Anderson (1972), a psychiatrist and mother of a brain-damaged child. Children with gross defects such as cerebral palsy or mental retardation are often treated with kindness and consider-ation, but those with minor defects—which may not be recognized as organic in origin—are often disruptive and tend to invite retaliation by parents, peers, teachers, and the public at large. Since these individuals do badly under stress, the organically determined behavioral disturbances are further compounded by their adverse reactions to a hostile environment. They run away from home, are truant from school, and develop feelings of guilt and unworthiness.

Most *adult* behavioral problems resulting from brain damage fall into one of two classes. A comparatively large number of brain-damaged individuals have a history of minimal brain dysfunction, whether developmental or acquired, arising in infancy or early childhood. Under sheltered conditions some find a niche in life suited to their level of competence, and adjust fairly well. Others do badly. Psychoses are more common in this group than in their siblings, and in addition some become drifters, alcoholics, or unsuccessful criminals, or do poorly professionally and domestically without displaying antisocial tendencies. Episodic dyscontrol is not uncommon, but it is sometimes difficult to uncover the true facts of the case because families of such people do their best to hide the situation. A common strategem is for them to deny that there is anything wrong, or that the attacks of rage are pathological or a matter for medical concern. Euphemisms are used to camouflage serious attacks on people or pets and wanton destruction of property. Spouse batterers and child abusers often admit only to "a short fuse" or "irritability," or they will say "I get nervous" or "I get uptight"—terms that scarcely do justice to some of the bloody encounters to which they refer. Denial is sometimes due to partial or total amnesia for what they did or said during violent incidents, and many are unconvinced until they actually see the physical damage they have wrought. Those whose violence is only verbal find it difficult to accept the victim's version of what they said during the attack.

The second group of adults consists of formerly normal individuals whose personality is sharply altered—almost always for the worse—by a brain insult, e.g., severe head injury, encephalitis, stroke, multiple sclerosis, Alzheimer's disease, slowly growing brain tumor, etc. Many such people are fully aware of their incapacity, but some—especially those who have frontal or parietal injuries—become euphoric and tend to deny their intellectual, emotional, and physical problems.

Episodic dyscontrol occurs in only a small proportion of people with head injuries, brain tumors, multiple sclerosis, and other organic conditions. An exception is encephalitis lethargica, which in the original epidemic produced a large crop of violent antisocial personality disorders. Today head injuries contribute more to intrafamilial violence than any other acquired condition in this group, as a result of chronic irritability and episodic dyscontrol.

Organic neurological disorders in the *victims* also play a part in intra-familial violence. Whereas the brain-damaged child in a favorable family environment often excites almost excessive devotion from the parents, it is also possible for an aggressive, destructive, hyperkinetic child to evoke antipathy and to invite abuse. This also applies to some epileptic children with behavioral problems and to children with learning disabilities caused by minimal brain damage. The fact that many brain-damaged children are sickly and somewhat helpless increases the risk of their being victimized. Needless to say, the interaction between a brain-damaged child and a parent who suffers from emotional dyscontrol can have dire results. A brain-damaged parent may incite violence at the hands of adolescent children, especially in social strata in which aggression is condoned. A mildly retarded wife or husband who cannot cope successfully with the complexities of life may incur the wrath of a normal spouse who does not realize the true state of affairs. A wife and mother who is aggressive because of unrecognized brain damage will sometimes provoke other members of the family to physical retaliation. There is also the problem of the masochistic or sadistic individual who deliberately or subconsciously prods a brain-damaged partner into violent behavior.

Another cause for friction, often unrecognized, is a mild degree of intellectual impairment such as is common after a head injury. The patient is told by a doctor that he or she has recovered and that there are no residual signs of damage. However, the patient knows that this is not so. Intellectual tasks are a little more difficult, memory is unreliable, mental and physical energy are somewhat reduced. There is less zest for life. Loud noises are insupportable, and headaches are common. Libido is often reduced. In adolescence there is usually a falling off of school work, which is a source of irritation and anxiety to the parents. The older patient often finds that his or her capacity to earn a living or advance in his or her profession is reduced. This leads to depression and anxiety except in those individuals who have had a severe frontal injury and are euphoric in consequence (Roberts, 1979). The consequent loss of earnings can have a domino effect on the rest of the family.

It is important for the therapist, the patient, and the family to recognize the presence of organic defects and to make what is often a difficult distinction between what is organic and what is functional. Postconcussional symptoms, for instance, are apt to seem functional, especially if neurological investigation has been negative, but in many such cases careful investigation by neuropsychological tests conducted by an expert will reveal an organic pattern of defects. Overlong persistence of postconcussional symptoms, however, may have a neurotic basis.

WHAT TO LOOK FOR

Cultural Factors

It is easier to identify pathological violence, as in the dyscontrol syndrome, for instance, when it constitutes a break in the life style of the patient and family than in strata of society in which violence is common and little thought of. Davis (1963), writing about the American scene says, ''The lower classes not uncommonly teach their children and adolescents to strike out with their fists or knives and to be certain to hit first. Boys and girls engage in free-for-all family encounters.'' In *The Courage of His Convictions,* Parker and Allerton (1962) report a habitual criminal's statement, ''As long as I can remember I have seen violence in use all around me, my mother hitting the children, my brothers and sisters all whacking their mother or other children, the man downstairs bashing his wife, and so on.'' Clearly, this behavior is part of a subculture, a means of expression, and in some cases a means of survival. It is essentially predatory. Scenes of general mayhem are less common in middle and upper-class families, though individual outbursts are not uncommon. In a violent subculture most of the combatants can control themselves *if they need to,* whereas in true dyscontrol, inhibitions are weak or absent. However, it is only too easy to fall into the trap of assuming that because a violent person comes from a violent home and belongs to a violent subculture, his or her violence is necessarily a cultural habit. It might be, and often is, biological in origin because some biological factors—such as head injuries, epilepsy, minimal brain dysfunction, and low IQ—are especially prevalent in the lower economic strata of society.

Violence in Antisocial Personality Disorders

A second type of violence, found at every social level, is the cold-blooded impulsive violence of the aggressive psychopath who uses physical violence without compunction to gain an objective. Such violence is usually carried out without anger and with a lack of foresight as to the consequences (Cleckley, 1976; Elliott, 1978). The physiological basis of this type of aggression is not known, but it is sometimes produced in a previously normal person by bilateral damage to the prefrontal lobes, and in children by diffuse damage to the basal ganglia and brain stem (as in encephalitis lethargica). In both monkeys and man bilateral prefrontal lesions can produce, in varying degrees, a change of personality. The patient becomes egocentric, incapable of affection, without conscience, lacking in insight, poor in external judgments, deficient in foresight, impulsive, unduly passive or highly aggressive, unreliable, untruthful, unable to learn from experience, lacking a sense of fear, prone to pathological intoxication with small quantities of alcohol and—occasionally—a liking for primitive and juvenile jokes (Elliott, 1978).

In many aggressive psychopaths, however, there is no history of physical trauma to the brain or other organic process, but there is a history of emotional deprivation in early life. There is microscopic, chemical, and electrophysiological evidence that in animals, including monkeys, isolation of babies from parents or peers can permanently interfere with the normal development of the brain and can produce an asocial adult whose behavior closely mimics that of the human psychopath—including abuse of its own young (Harlow & Mears, 1979). Emotional deprivation and isolation seems to retard the maturation of the neurological bases of social adaptation and emotional development in small children. It can also depress the growth hormone and produce "psychosocial dwarfism"; growth resumes when the child is transplanted to favorable surroundings.

Psychopathic behavior, whether dating from childhood or occurring in a previously normal adult following a brain insult such as a head injury, is essentially infantile, and when linked to a good intelligence and personal charm can have a devastating effect on family life and on society.

Psychotic Hostility

A third form of violence is the "acting out" episodes that sometimes occur in the course of various mental disorders such as borderline syndromes, typical and atypical schizophrenias, manic depressive psychosis, and the catathymic crises of passive-aggressive personalities. From the practical point of view, though the behavior of the patient when "acting out" superficially resembles the explosive behavior of the episodic dyscontrol syndrome of organic origin, the patient usually exhibits conspicuous psychopathology between attacks of violence.

THE ORGANIC EPISODIC DYSCONTROL SYNDROME OF EXPLOSIVE RAGE

This account is based on a neurological review of 286 private patients who had a history of violence in the home. Over 90% were Caucasian and middle or upper class. The great majority were not delinquent in so far as they had not been taken to court on account of their violence, though many deserved to be. Overt psychotics, core psychopaths, border-line cases, mentally retarded persons, and those whose violence was exclusively drug related were excluded from the study.

What these people had in common was a history of repeated episodes of explosive rage in response to minor provocations or, in some cases, no provocation at all. The attacks resulted in assaults on people and animals, destruction of property, and in some instances verbal abuse that was almost as destructive in a social sense as physical brutality. At one end of the scale were many who fell within the limits of intermittent explosive disorder as defined in DSM III (the Diagnostic and Statistical Manual of the American Psychiatric Association, Volume 3); between their attacks of rage, which were entirely out of character, they were not overly impulsive or aggressive, and they were certainly not psychotic, but during the episodes there was a total change of personality, voice, and manner. At the other end of the scale were those who exhibited mild cognitive defects, neurotic symptoms, or personality disorders between their rages, but whose violence was the predominant problem. Such cases were located along the axis of a continuum running between intermittent explosive disorder at one end and overt psychiatric illness at the other. In all cases, physical violence was primitive—gouging, kicking, clawing, spitting, biting—and the attacks were carried out so swiftly and with such great force that the victim was hard put to escape. Verbal assaults were characterized by unwonted profanity and obscenity. The attacks usually tapered off within 5 to 60 minutes leaving a sense of exhaustion and sometimes a patchy amnesia for what had been done or said. Remorse usually followed within a few hours and in a few cases led to attempts at suicide.

According to DSM III the intermittent explosive disorder is "very rare" but it might be more accurate to say that patients with this disorder rarely seek medical or psychiatric help because most of them seem to think that what they call a bad temper is their own affair and not a matter for medical, much less psychiatric, interference. This attitude persists even in people whose career or marriage has been spoiled by their behavior. Some of the subjects in the study had sought professional help and not received it—a common event in the experience of Mark and Ervin (1970). A middle-aged engineer lost not only several jobs but no less than three wives because of his violence. The parting shot from the third wife was that he should go and see a psychiatrist. This he resolutely refused to do but was persuaded to see a neurologist, whom he regarded as the lesser of two evils. Investigation revealed well-marked cognitive and motor defects dating from childhood and consistent with a diagnosis of minimal brain dysfunction.

In some, the dyscontrol appears to be relative rather than absolute in that the affected individuals are often able to control themselves in the presence of strangers, therapists, **or p**olicemen, but not at home. Even at home rage excited by an altercati**on w**ith a child or wife may be directed not at the individual but at the furniture, or the family pet, or the windows. Many report that they *can* control themselves up to a point—sufficient to walk away from a confrontation—but if the rage gets beyond this point, ''I can't stop it.'' Because of self-control such individuals exercise in public, physicians do not often see an attack and may underestimate how fierce it can be. It is a salutary learning experience. In one recent case, it took five large policemen and a ward orderly 20 minutes to subdue a lightly built man age 21. Between attacks he appeared normal, but it was difficult to avoid the conclusion that in this episode he was indeed temporarily insane. Consider also the case of a highly controlled and ordinarily gentle Quaker lady of 65. During a social occasion she turned on her husband for no apparent reason and poured forth a stream of obscene vituperation, much of which was obscured by animal-like snarls and growls, foam lightly flecking her lips. After a few painful minutes, shaking with rage, she turned slowly and went out of the room to come back ten minutes later, sit down quietly, and say, ''I am sorry.'' Such attacks had occurred at irregular intervals since a severe head injury at the age of 19. Her husband said that doctors had never believed him when he described these episodes to them because they knew her to be a kindly and refined woman of high intelligence. His complaint is echoed by many battered wives and some battered husbands who have vainly sought medical help or police protection.

In many cases there was a history of familial violence—physical, verbal, or both. It can be difficult to get accurate facts about relatives and ancestors in this mobile society, but in those instances where the record appeared to be well substantiated it was clear that not all children of a violent parent become violent themselves. Some remember the parental battles with horror but others shrug off their own violent episodes with the excuse that ''I guess it runs in the family.'' In several pedigrees, however, it was found that explosive behavior had affected about half the siblings in each of two or three generations, and in one case, four generations. Davenport (1915) found this to be the case in a group of delinquent girls whose explosive behavior had contributed to their crimes. He found that only half the siblings in each generation were violent and concluded that in these cases explosive rage was a dominant trait whether it appeared in epileptics, psychotics, or otherwise normal individuals. It seems that while violent behavior as a way of life is often learned, liability to episodic dyscontrol can be inherited. In nine cases of this series it appeared to be an inherited trait in people without overt organic disease or psychopathology.

In this study, 102 people, previously regarded as equable, developed explosive behavior following physical damage to the brain (e.g., trauma, stroke, tumor, Alzheimer's disease, multiple sclerosis, encephalitis, encephalopathy) or as a temporary episode resulting from hypoglycemia. Eighteen of the remaining 184 had no detectable evidence of physical disease, and 119 had signs of minimal brain dysfunction. Forty-seven had epilepsy, and another 60 had seizures as a complication of minimal brain dysfunction (MBD), head injury, etc. So, next to explosive rage, seizures were the most common symptom, having been present in 37.5% of the entire series, a prevalence some 60 times greater than in the general population.

Epilepsy

In most cases involving epilepsy the attacks were infrequent and mild. Convulsions and dramatic attacks of unconsciousness were rare and only seven had had grand mal attacks. Most of the episodes were classified as complex partial seizures, a term which includes temporal lobe epilepsy and psychomotor epilepsy—brief attacks marked by an alteration in the quality and content of consciousness, often associated with inappropriate and maladaptive behavior. It is not enough to ask whether the patient had seizures or convulsions or attacks of unconsciousness because many will truthfully deny any knowledge of them. They do not realize that the strange experiences they have had from time to time were psychomotor seizures but are apt to attribute them to "nerves," hypoglycemia, and so on. Temporal lobe epileptics are particularly prone to describe their symptoms at great length and enormous detail in written reports that sometimes do more to obscure than to illuminate the diagnosis unless the physician knows that graphorrhea is not uncommon in temporal lobe epileptics. Individual attacks often consist of such complex and essentially psychic disturbances as brief mental confusion, delusions, hallucinations (olfactory, visual, auditory), brief changes in affect such as fear, depression, elation, and occasionally anger, or disturbances of memory or ideation, dreamy states, double consciousness, depersonalization, slowing or acceleration of ambient sounds, altered time perception, a sense that things look different, and so on. Automatisms may exist on their own or be linked to any of the above. These include smacking of the lips, swallowing or chewing movements, water drinking, spitting, inappropriate laughter or weeping, cursive attacks, disrobing in public, gestural automatisms such as head scratching, nose rubbing, brushing dust off clothes, slapping the thigh, etc., and inappropriate erotic activity. Ictal rage can occur, but it is generally considered to be rare. Postictal violence and interictal episodic dyscontrol are more common. There is no evidence that an epileptic attack can consist of well-coordinated planned aggressive behavior directed towards a distinct and gainful purpose. Autonomic disturbances which often accompany general and focal seizures sometimes occur more or less on their own. They include brief episodes of sweating, cyanosis (from disordered breathing), blushing, pallor, tachycardia, piloerection, and—of course—incontinence of urine and/or feces. An excellent account of these and other forms of complex partial seizures has been provided by Daly (1975).

Minimal Brain Dysfunction

By far the most common neurological finding in this series was the syndrome of minimal brain dysfunction (MBD) (Wender, 1971; Cantwell, 1975; Millichap, 1978; Pincus & Tucker, 1978). It had generally been obvious in childhood, and fragments of the syndrome had persisted in adolescence and adult life (Wood, 1976). For instance, a hyperkinetic, clumsy, dyslexic child who suffered from severe temper tantrums ended up as an adult who still had some difficulty in reading and slight manual clumsiness, and was also liable to intermittent rages.

Minimal brain dysfunction is not a theoretical concept. The symptoms are due to a heterogenous collection of neuropathological conditions, developmental and acquired. Developmental defects—which are sometimes familial—include small vascular malformations, dense collections of glial cells in areas where they don't belong (as in the cortex and white matter), ectopic groups of abnormal-looking nerve cells in the white matter, and multiple patches of cortical dysplasia in which the architecture of cortical layers is grossly disturbed. The brain often looks normal on the surface, and it requires microscopic examination of serial sections of the entire brain to identify the defects, which are usually multiple. This prodigious task is seldom undertaken, and the result of such an examination in a case of familial dyslexia, published by Galaburda and Kemper (1979), is therefore important because it demonstrated multiple patches of cortical dysplasia in various parts of one cerebral hemisphere in a boy who was dyslexic, clumsy, epileptic, and emotionally stable.

The most common cause of acquired defects is hypoxia during or immediately following birth or caused by *prolonged* convulsions in early infancy. Brief febrile convulsions do not qualify. Examination of the brain in 55 epileptics by Margerrison and Corsellis (1966) revealed multiple scars in almost all cases, the most numerous being in the hippocampus, followed in order of frequency by the cerebellum, amygdala, thalamus, and cerebral cortex. Other acquired lesions are scars and loss of neurons from head injuries and infections, and porencephalic cysts of undetermined origin. Arrested hydrocephalus without external evidence thereof is sometimes found by pneumoencephalography or, more recently, by CT scan.

It is often impossible to identify with certainty the event that caused the damage in a single case, because there is nothing in the history to give a lead, but it must be remembered that the infant brain can be permanently damaged by malnutrition, by toxins such as lead, and by illnesses such as encephalitis, which masquerades as ordinary influenza. Another cause is unrecorded trauma caused by falls, by deliberate blows to the head by a parent, and even by violently shaking an infant held by the shoulders, which causes no outward signs of damage but can give rise to intracerebral and subdural hemorrhages.

The early symptoms of MBD may be very slight. During the first week or two the baby may be excessively sleepy, or sleepless, or there may be an inverted sleep rhythm. Such babies are often prone to colic and scream incessantly; some are unnaturally quiet. As they grow older the mother will perhaps notice that they are not "cuddly" and seek to avoid physical contact. They may be inert or hyperkinetic in infancy and childhood. Some of the milestones of development may be deferred. Severe tantrums are common. The child is often clumsy, maladroit in the handling of toys or dolls. Later on there come scholastic and behavioral problems at school; the child does not live up to expectations as judged by his or her general intelligence. Patchy cognitive defects are identified, in the absence of mental retardation, and specific learning problems appear, notably in reading, writing, arithmetic, or spelling, or in sequential memory (inability to learn the sequence of a simple poem or to remember the order of the letters of the alphabet or months of the year). The child may exhibit spotty defects in motor ability with good athletic capacity for some tasks and none in others. He or she may fail to ride a bicycle or to jump rope or hit a ball with a bat or to catch a ball. At a later date, some people are never able to learn to dance, however hard they try, while others have difficulty in swinging a club to hit a golf ball. Their efforts to do so are often grotesque. It is characteristic of MBD that both the cognitive and the motor defects are usually spotty and stand out against a background of normal capacity in related functions. Unlike the general clumsiness of MBD, these defects are examples of apraxia and/or agnosia (Gubbay, 1975). Sometimes there are subtle disturbances of sensation and of the reflexes. The persistence of nocturnal bed wetting beyond the age of six is very common in boys. Though it is often influenced by emotional situations, the underlying defect is usually a maturational lag in the development of the autonomic nervous control of the bladder and sphincters.

In addition to obviously neurological problems many children with MBD show characteristic psychological and behavioral disturbances, which often dominate the scene. They include impulsiveness, a short attention span, poverty of abstract thought, imperceptiveness in social and other situations, poor judgment, lack of insight, inability to distinguish between figure and ground, left/right disorientation, direction agnosia with a capacity for getting lost (and later on, inability to read a map). Some display antisocial features—lack of conscience, no sense of guilt, little empathy with others, senseless lying, and total unreliability. Some appear to be wholly insensitive to punishment.

A more detailed description of the outstanding features of adult minimal brain dysfunction is published elsewhere (Elliott, in press).

Prospective and retrospective studies have shown that while some people with MBD find a useful niche in adult life, or even achieve distinguished positions (e.g., Beethoven), others do not. Those with childhood MBD are more likely to suffer psychiatric disorders than their normal siblings. Others simply fail to live up to their capacity and add to the pool of professional failures and social misfits. A damaged brain is more prone than a normal one to give incorrect solutions, a principle best illustrated by the dramatic transformation of the personality, always for the worse, which can follow *appropriately situated* brain damage in a previously normal person. Examples of this are given elsewhere (Elliott, 1978).

Evidence of MBD was found in 41% of the 286 violent people studied, and this is probably an underestimate because when the study started 10 years ago we did not always ask the right questions. We also used the traditional adult type of neurological examination instead of the expanded version which is necessary to uncover the subtle neurological signs and symptoms of the condition. Moreover, at that time the CT scan was not available. When it did become available, it disclosed structural lesions, many of them unexpected, in no less than 41% of 148 cases.

Head Injury

Severe head injuries followed by a period of unconsciousness lasting 7 days, or multiple small injuries, often give rise to intellectual impairment, change of personality, and explosive behavior, and thus contribute to violence in the family. Most severe closed injuries produce damage to the undersurface of the frontal lobe and anterior part of the temporal lobes, irrespective of what part of the head is hit; microscopic damage is also found in the brain stem. This is to say, the damage usually involves parts of the brain that are concerned, among other things, with the expression and regulation of emotions, including control of aggressive impulses.

It has been estimated that every year in the United States about three million individuals suffer a head injury and of these 200,000 survive but suffer permanent brain damage. About 10% of them may be expected to suffer from episodic dyscontrol in addition to various degrees of cognitive, perceptual, and other neurological problems (Roberts, 1979). In children, severe head injuries are particularly liable to produce permanent and serious disorders of personality, often with relatively less impact on intellectual capacity. "Common antisocial trends included unrestrained aggressiveness, destructiveness, quarrelsomeness, cruelty to younger children and animals, lying and stealing. Their whole personality is essentially egocentric and self interested with total disregard for the welfare of others'' (Blau, 1936). Even mild head injuries in which the patient was rendered unconscious for only a few hours can produce subtle changes of personality at all ages. The family notices that the afflicted member has never been quite the same since the accident. In some the changes are far from subtle; a pleasant man with a peaceful disposition was knocked unconscious for about 2 days, after which he made what seemed to be a complete recovery except that within a few months he found that his tolerance for alcohol was diminished in a most unfortunate way. After not more than two pints of beer, he might become extremely combative and would attack members of his family or total strangers with great ferocity. During these spells he showed none of the usual features of drunkenness but became a changed personality and a very dangerous one at that. On two occasions he killed total strangers. The attacks were followed by total amnesia for the event. When he stopped drinking the attacks ceased. This abnormal response to small quantities of alcohol is seen in other organic conditions of the brain, notably in those who also suffer from episodic dyscontrol without the aid of alcohol. In them, small ''social'' quantities of alcohol are apt to trigger off attacks of uncontrollable rage.

OTHER SOURCES OF EPISODIC DYSCONTROL

Also related to violent behavior are brain tumors, stroke, encephalitis, multiple sclerosis, Alzheimer's disease, and rare conditions such as cardiorespiratory arrest, Huntington's chorea, and hypoglycemia, examples of which account for 51 cases in this series. The tumors are particularly interesting in this context because of the light they throw on the pathophysiology of episodic explosive rage. Thirteen patients had small tumors, 12 in areas in or near the midline of the cerebral hemispheres and involving the phylogenetically ancient limbic system or the hypothalamus. That is, they all involved ancient structures that are relics of the reptilian and neomammalian brain. None involved the neocortex, which is in line with Bard's 1928 discovery that damage to the neocortex does not produce the syndrome of explosive rage in experimental animals. It is sometimes argued that explosive behavior in brain tumor cases is really a reaction to pain, fear, or physical disability, but in these 13 cases this was not so. In five cases explosive behavior started months *after* the successful surgical removal of the tumor, probably as a result of surgical scarring. In another three, explosive rage was the first symptom occurring before the onset of headache, mental confusion, or physical incapacity. It should be added that in children small benign tumors of the pons, which is also an ancient structure, can give rise to explosive rage and change of personality as an early symptom.

Encephalitis lethargica provided another dramatic example of the link between organic disease, psychopathic behavior, and violence. During the world epidemic of this disease in the second decade of the present century, various psychological sequelae appeared in at least 30% of the children it attacked: "These children are destructive and impulsive. Impulses are immediately translated into actions. Inhibition and fear of consequence are lacking. They steal, lie, destroy property, set fires and commit sex offenses. They do not try to avoid detection and claim that they cannot help their conduct. They are indifferent to punishment. When they express remorse this does not modify their behavior" (Bender, 1962). The main brunt of this disease was on the upper brain stem and basal ganglia. It is rare today but other forms of encephalitis occasionally produce similar though less severe disorders of personality and behavior and, like encephalitis lethargica, may cause little impairment of intellectual capacity. In this series there were 13 cases of encephalitis or encephalopathy.

METABOLIC DISORDERS

The most common metabolic disorder involving behavior and affecting family life is the premenstrual tension syndrome. Some women experience emotional dyscontrol, with or without other symptoms, mainly in the week prior to menstruation. The attacks are usually marked by depression, paranoia, irrational thinking and irritability, and sometimes by typical uncontrolled fits of rage during which they are apt to attack their male consort or the children, physically or verbally. Morton (1953) found that 62% of violent crimes committed by a group of women prisoners had occurred in the premenstrual week and only 2% at the end of menstruation. This trend was confirmed by Dalton (1964, 1979). In France the syndrome is sometimes accepted as an extenuating circumstance in crimes of violence and recently this plea has been successfully used in two cases in Britain (Lancet, 1981).

Many women are aware of minor degrees of premenstrual tension but are not violent. They feel depressed and, as one put it, "In those few days I hate everybody and in particular I hate myself for being so bitchy." Even when the violence is verbal rather than physical it leads to quarrels and sometimes to physical retaliation on the part of the male.

Another metabolic disorder that can trigger dyscontrol is a sudden fall of blood sugar, which can be functional, or due to insulin overdosage or excessive secretion of insulin by the pancreas. This usually causes sweating and a sense of weakness; in extreme cases the patient may lose consciousness and have a convulsion. Occasionally, however, it does none of these things but gives rise to bizarre behavior that is sometimes violent. The violence may continue for as much as a half an hour, and much destruction can be caused. Though Wilder (1947) assembled a formidable bibliography, including references to instances of intrafamilial strife, attacks of extreme violence are less common than unpredictable irritability and lack of judgment. Sometimes attacks of rage are triggered by hypoglycemia in somebody who turns out to have psychomotor epilepsy or a brain tumor, or cerebral arteriosclerosis, so that the diagnosis is not completely established solely by the demonstration of hypoglycemia induced by a 5-hour glucose tolerance test.

Reactive hypoglycemia can also be caused in normal subjects by drinking alcohol on an empty stomach if, for example, several drinks are taken in the evening after a long day of physical exercise and little to eat. It is particularly likely to occur if the alcohol is combined with sugar-containing soft drinks (as in "gin and tonic"). This combination can induce a sense of extreme weakness with a fall of blood pressure, or it may trigger rage.

THE PREVENTION OF EXPLOSIVE RAGE

Individual violence has so many origins and such a wide neurological substrate that no single drug can be expected to be universally successful. The same applies to psychosurgery, which is seldom necessary today. Nevertheless, it would be inaccurate to say, as some do, that there is no drug for violence. It is more correct to say that although there is no drug that can *cure* violence in a definitive way, the last 30 years have seen slow but definite progress in the *symptomatic* control of some types of aggressive behavior. Those who remember the destructive interictal behavior of many epileptics in the days when only phenobarbitone and bromides were available will recall the pleasure with which we observed that the effect of Dilantin on behavior was sometimes as dramatic as its anticonvulsant action, and this holds true today. Carbamezapine is also successful in many epileptics and in some nonepileptics. In the 1950s the phenothiazines brought a measure of tranquility to mental hospitals. Kline (1962) reported that prior to the use of major tranquilizers in the Rockland State Hospital, 8,000 windowpanes were broken in a single year, requiring the attention of three full-time glaziers, but by 1960 only 1,900 were broken annually. The lesser tranquilizers have their place, too, as do the amphetamines and methylphenidate in the treatment of the hyperactive syndrome and the violence that may go with it. Lithium is an effective drug for many unipolar and bipolar affective states and also, in some cases, for the control of episodic rage in the absence of overt affective psychoses. A recent addition to the list is propranolol (Inderal), which has proved useful in the prevention of explosive rage in cases of head injury, epilepsy, and other organic disorders in adults (Elliott, 1977; Yudofsky, Williams, & Gorman, 1981) and in children prone to explosive tantrums.

Although these advances ease the problem of the therapists to some extent, the violent individual and his or her family continue to need support. It is wise to make provision for a ''hot line'' and other means of access to professional help at short notice for patients who feel they are on the brink of losing control. Both the family and the patient must learn to break off confrontations before they become uncontrollable, for example, by leaving the room (though *not* by going out in the car where they may vent their anger on other motorists). Eye-to-eye contact should be avoided and it should be remembered that ''a soft answer turneth away wrath.''

The management of the violent patient in hospitals and institutions has been well described by Lion (1972), who pays appropriate attention to the role of organic disorders. One of the problems in dealing with some violent people is that they are impulsive and easily frustrated, so if the treatment they are receiving does not work immediately, they often forsake the doctor and seek another, and eventually become sufficiently disillusioned to refuse to take either advice or medication. Nevertheless, much may be done for intelligent and cooperative patients who really want to gain control of themselves and who will accept the fact that it may take a little time before a suitable medication can be found. After prolonged psychotherapy many understand some of the reasons for their explosive outbursts, but continue to have them. Pharmaceutical intervention is then necessary. Many have expressed relief when told after neurological investigation that their dyscontrol attacks are partly a result of physical defects in their inhibitory circuits. The words "brain damage" should be sedulously avoided. The phamacological treatment of personality disorders and delinquents has been well reviewed by Kellner (1978), and the prevention of dyscontrol by propranolol is discussed by Elliott (1977).

The use of alcohol is to be discouraged because organic cases are particularly liable to pathological intoxication and are easily triggered into rage by quite small quantities if they happen to be in an irritable phase.

Phenothiazines and barbiturates are best avoided in organic cases as they can trigger explosive rage, in contrast to their tranquilizing effect in functional neuroses and psychoses. Smoking "pot," on the other hand, is reported by many patients to be the quickest way of banishing aggressive feelings and avoiding violent outbursts. Other street drugs should be avoided entirely and at all times, particularly while legitimate pharmaceuticals are being used to prevent aggressive behavior. (Individuals refusing to cooperate were excluded from the present study.) For the irritability and rages in the premenstrual tension syndrome Meprobamate is useful in mild cases. (It has also been used successfully for the control of the lethal intraspecies violence of tropical fighting fish.) Dalton (1979) reports that severe cases are greatly helped by the administration of *natural* progesterone by suppository or injection in the week preceding menstruation. Synthetic varieties are ineffective. Premenstrual hypoglycemia may provide an additional stimulus for irritability and should be treated appropriately when found.

SUMMARY

Of the many ways in which neurological disorders can contribute to intrafamilial violence—some of which are described—none is more distinct than the syndrome of explosive rage, which is one variety of the episodic dyscontrol syndrome.

This paper reports the neurological findings in 286 patients with a history of repeated intrafamilial violence against spouse, children, pets, or property. Overt psychotics, core psychopaths, retarded persons, and drug addicts were arbitrarily excluded from the study. In 184 cases the violence dated from tantrums in early childhood. In the remainder it started after an identifiable brain insult, such as a head injury or encephalitis, in a formerly equable person.

In two-thirds of the cases, the patient was judged to be psychiatrically unremarkable between attacks of rage, which perhaps explains the forebearance shown to many of them by members of the family and their success in evading court action. One-third presented a variety of additional psychiatric symptoms, which ran in a continuum through neuroses to borderline syndromes.

The neurological examination was directed especially to uncovering evidence of temporal lobe seizures and the syndrome of minimal brain dysfunction in adults. Clinical examination was buttressed by electroencephalography, CT scans (in 148 patients), five-hour glucose tolerance tests, and neuropsychological tests for evidence of organic disorder when they were deemed essential.

Objective evidence of developmental or acquired defects was found in 94%. The most common abnormality was minimal brain dysfunction (41%). The most common *symptom* apart from episodic dyscontrol was complex partial seizures, which had occurred at some time in the life of 30%.

In many the attacks were not recognized as epileptic because of their subtle form and rare occurrence.

The high percentage of abnormalities found in this group is partly attributable to biased selection on the part of the referring physicians, partly to the use of the CT scan (which disclosed many unsuspected structural abnormalities), and partly to pains taken to uncover MBD in adults and adolescents. The conventional adult form of neurological examination is largely insensitive to the subtle signs of the heterogeneous developmental and acquired defects that constitute minimal brain dysfunction.

Attention is drawn to the value of nontranquilizing drugs in the treatment of episodic dyscontrol. They include anticonvulsants such as the phenytoins and carbamezapine; stimulants such as the amphetamines and methylphenidate; propranolol; lithium; and, for the premenstrual tension syndrome, *natural* progesterone.

In view of the high prevalence of organic defects in this atypical sample, there is need for an investigation of the neurological status of an unselected group of spouse batterers and child abusers with particular attention to forms of organic brain impairments that are not immediately obvious but that are known to be capable of interfering with emotional control and social adaptation.

REFERENCES

Anderson, C. *Society pays. The high cost of minimal brain dysfunction in America.* New York: Walker, 1972.

Andrulonis, P.A., Glueck, B.C., Strobel C.F., Vogel, M.G., Shapiro, A.L., & Aldridge, D. Organic brain dysfunction in the borderline syndrome. *Psychiatric Clinics of North America,* 1980, *4,* 47–65.

Bach-Y-Rita, G., Lion, J.R., Climent, C.F., & Ervin, F.R. Episodic dyscontrol: A study of 130 violent patients. *American Journal of Psychiatry,* 1971, *127,* 1473–1478.

Bard, P. Diencephalic mechanism for the expression of rage. *American Journal of Physiology,* 1928, *89,* 490–515.

Bellak, L. (Ed.). *Psychiatric aspects of minimal brain dysfunction in adults.* New York: Grune & Stratton, 1979.

Bender, L., & Neal, J.B. (Eds.). *Encephalitis—a clinical study.* New York: Grune & Stratton, 1962.

Blau, A. Mental changes following trauma in children. *Archives of Neurology,* 1936, *35,* 723–730.

Cantwell, D.P. (Ed.). *The hyperactive child.* New York: Spectrum, 1975.

Cleckley, H. *The mask of sanity* (5th ed.). St. Louis: Mosby, 1976.

Dalton, K. *The premenstrual syndrome.* London: William Heinemann Medical Books, 1964.

Dalton, K. *Once a month: The premenstrual syndrome.* Pomona, Calif.: Hunter House, 1979.

Daly, D.D. Ictal clinical manifestations of complex partial seizures. Chap. 4 in J.K. Penry & D.D. Daley (Eds.), *Advances in Neurology,* Vol. II. New York: Raven Press, 1975.

Davenport, C.B. The feebly inherited: Violent temper and its inheritance. *Journal of Nervous and Mental Disease,* 1915, *42,* 593–628.

Davis, W.A. Child rearing in the class structure of American society. In M.S. Sussman (Ed.), *Source book of marriage and the family.* Boston: Houghton Mifflin, 1963.

Elliott, F.A. Propranolol for the control of belligerent behavior following acute brain damage. *Annals of Neurology,* 1977, *1,* 489–496.

Elliott, F.A. Neurological aspects of antisocial behavior. Chap. 8 in W.H. Reid (Ed.), *The psychopath: A comprehensive study of antisocial disorders and behaviors.* New York: Brunner/Mazel, 1978.

Elliott, F.A. Neurological findings in adult minimal brain dysfunction and the dyscontrol syndrome. *Journal of Nervous and Mental Disease,* Special Issue on Atypical Psychoses, in press.

Galaburda, A.M., & Kemper, T.L. Cytoarchitectonic abnormalities in developmental dyslexia. *Annals of Neurology,* 1979, *6,* 96–101.

Gubbay, S.S. *The clumsy child. A study of developmental apraxia and agnosic ataxia.* Philadelphia: Saunders, 1975.

Hare, R.P., & Schalling, D. (Eds.). *Psychopathic Behavior.* New York: Wiley, 1978.

Harlow, H.F., & Mears, C. *The human model: Primate perspectives.* Washington, D.C.: Winston, 1979.

Healy, W. & Bronner, A.F. *New light on delinquency and its treatment.* New Haven, Conn.: Yale University Press, 1936.

Hill, J.D., & Watterson D. EEG studies of psychopathic personalities. *Journal of Neurology and Psychiatry,* 1942, *5,* 47–52.

Horowitz, H.A. Psychiatric casualties of minimal brain dysfunction in adolescence. *Annals of Adolescent Psychiatry*, 1982, *9*, 275–294.

Kellner, R. Drug treatment of personality disorders of delinquents. Chap. 10 in W.H. Reid (Ed.), *The psychopath*. New York: Brunner/Mazel, 1978.

Kline, M. Drugs are the greatest medical advance in the history of psychiatry. *New Medical Material*, 1962, *6*, 49–52.

Lancet. *The premenstrual syndrome. (editorial)*, December 19, 1981, *ii*, 1393–1394.

Lion, J.R. *Evaluation and management of the violent patient*. Springfield, Ill.: Charles C Thomas, 1972.

Margerrison, J., & Corsellis, J.A. Epilepsy in the temporal lobes. A clinical and neuropathological study. *Brain*, 1966, *89*, 499–528.

Mark, V.H., & Ervin, F.R. *Violence and the brain*. New York: Harper & Row, 1970.

Mednick, S., & Christiansen, K.O. *Biosocial bases on criminal behavior*. New York: Gardner Press, 1977.

Millichap, J.G. *The hyperactive child and minimal brain dysfunction*. Chicago: Yearbook Medical Publications, 1978.

Monroe, R.R. *Episodic behavioral disorders*. Cambridge, Mass.: Harvard University Press, 1970.

Moore, M. Encephalographic studies of schizophrenics (Dementia Praecox). *American Journal of Psychiatry*, 1933, *12*, 801–810.

Morton, J.H., Additon, H., Addison, R.G., Hunt, L., & Sullivan, B. A clinical study of premenstrual tension. *American Journal of Obstetrics & Gynecology*, 1953, *65*, 1182–1191.

Parker, T., & Allerton, K. *The courage of his convictions*. London: Hutchinson, 1962.

Pincus, J., & Tucker, G.J. *Behavioral neurology* (2nd ed.). New York: Oxford University Press, 1978.

Reid, W.H. (Ed.). *The psychopath: A comprehensive study of antisocial disorders and behaviors*. New York: Brunner/Mazel, 1978.

Roberts, A.H. *Severe accidental head injury*. London: MacMillan Press, 1979.

Thompson, G.N. *The psychopathic criminal and delinquent*. Springfield, Ill.: Charles C Thomas, 1953.

Wender, P.H. *Minimal brain dysfunction in children*. New York: Wiley Inter-Sciences, 1971.

Wilder, J. Sugar metabolism in its relation to criminology. In R.M. Lindner & R.V. Seliger (Eds.), *Handbook of correctional psychology*. New York. Philosophical Library, 1947.

Wood, D.R., Reimherr, W., Wender, P.H., & Johnson G.E. Diagnosis and treatment of minimal brain dysfunction in adults. *Archives of General Psychiatry*, 1976, *33*, 1453–1460.

Yeudall, L.T., & Fromm-Rauch, D. Neuropsychological impairments in various psychopathological populations. In J. Gruzelier & P. Flor-Henry (Eds.), *Hemisphere asymmetries of function in psychopathology*. Amsterdam: Elsevier/North Holland Biomedical Press, 1979.

Yudofsky, S., Williams, D., & Gorman, J. Propranolol in the treatment of rage and violent behavior in patients with chronic brain syndromes. *American Journal of Psychiatry*, 1981, *132*, 218–220.

4. The Dynamics of Rage between the Sexes in a Bonded Relationship

Herb Goldberg, Ph.D.
Licensed Psychologist
Los Angeles, California

Four

THE ACCUMULATION OF RAGE IN INTIMATE, BONDED, heterosexual relationships is built-in, inevitable, and in direct proportion to the extent of the man's ''masculine'' defenses and the woman's ''feminine'' defenses. It is a paradoxical and painful irony that the more classically romantic the relationship is at its onset, the more the phenomenon of rage building up holds true. At the same time, self-hate grows in the man and the woman who believe they are in a ''wonderful'' relationship that is supposed to feel good but they cannot seem to make it work.

To understand this buildup of rage, we need to look at the defensive processes involved in the gender conditioning we term masculinity and femininity. Traditionally, femininity involves a number of basic areas of repression. Little girls are taught to repress their sexuality (it's okay to be cuddly, but not ''horny''); to repress autonomy and power (it's not okay to be too strong or independent); to repress anger (''to be sugar and spice and everything nice''); and to repress their assertiveness (feminine women are supposed to be easy to get along with).

All of these are, of course, inauthentic or defensive responses. She has her anger, her willfulness, her strivings for autonomy, her ''horniness,'' and her needs for power and control. All of these are, however, more or less disguised and denied in the name of being feminine; and, instead they emerge and erupt indirectly or passively. Only at some later point— when the relationship has collapsed—do they become overt.

Likewise, masculinity is a set of defenses against dependency, emotionalism in general, vulnerability, passivity, absence of sexuality, fear, etc. A ''real'' man validates himself as ''masculine'' if he doesn't really need anybody, never lets emotions interfere with his responses, is "afraid of nothing," rarely tires, is always decisive, knows what to do and how to take charge, and is sexually always ready and able to perform "well."

Classically, romance is the process of a man and woman falling in love with each other's defenses, initially feeling rescued by the other and then coming to hate each other for the rigidity that underlies the defenses and for the belief that their growth is being blocked by the other person.

She is drawn to his "strength," "independence," assertion ("take-charge" quality), aggression ("he's not afraid of anybody"), sexuality (he's a "real man"), his drive and ambition, his rationality (he's so smart, so logical, he knows "everything"). Later in the relationship, however, she comes to resent him for these very same qualities and she begins to reinterpret them as follows: his independence becomes "He doesn't need me"; his assertiveness becomes "He tries to control me"; his sexuality becomes "I feel like he uses me"; his aggression becomes "His temper scares me"; and his rational, logical mind becomes "He's cold. He doesn't feel anything. He's always analyzing and intellectualizing."

Likewise, he is initially drawn to her emotionality ("She's so sensitive"); her compliance ("She's so easy to get along with"); her lack of overt aggression ("She doesn't have an angry bone in her body. She gets along with everyone"); her "sexual purity" ("Sex is special to her—she won't go to bed with just anybody"); and her dependence ("She really needs me").

Later, he comes to react to her dependency as if it were childlike smothering. Her emotionality becomes "She's irrational" and "I can't reason with her," or even "She's crazy"; her "sexual purity" becomes "She's frigid; I always feel like she's doing me a favor when we have sex, I never know when she really wants it"; her compliance becomes "She's boring" or "I don't know what she really wants"; and her repressed aggression becomes "She always tries to make me the bad guy."

Furthermore, rage builds up as they come to see each other as blocks to personal growth. She comes to blame him for not "allowing her" to be independent, assertive, sexual, and strong. He comes to feel that she only sees him as a provider and protector and won't allow him to expose his fear, his vulnerability, his desire to "let go" of ambition and his success drive, or to acknowledge his sexual anxiety and his needs and confusion. In short, he comes to feel she won't "let him" be a person.

He fears she won't love him if he's weak. She fears he won't love her if she's strong. Both, therefore, come to feel that "I can't be real around my partner. I feel trapped."

Conflict resolution between the two is difficult or impossible, in proportion to the degree of their gender polarization. First, they have been taught and have come to believe that love equals harmony; and a "bad" relationship is one where there is fighting and differences. Second, she has a tendency to deny her anger and aggression and to see herself as only wanting "peace" and "love." Her repressed aggression and assertion causes her to see herself as his victim. She wants to change *him* to improve the relationship. His masculine sense of being "in charge" and "responsible" tends to weigh him down with an excessive sense of guilt when things go wrong. Third, he has learned that his role means that he is to be her protector because she is essentially fragile. Therefore, he tends to withhold crucial information about his feelings and himself for fear that she won't be able to "take it." Likewise, her self image of being "nice" prevents her from showing him the full force of her strength and anger. She is also unduly fearful of his aggression.

In other words, they have learned that man-woman relationships are supposed to be loving if they're "normal" or good. They have never been taught to fight things out openly, or to focus objectively on their own parts in creating the conflict situations and problems without blame, guilt, or judgment. Instead, she tends to blame and feel victimized. He tends to withdraw, then overreact with rage and then guilt, and then to try to "make up," but with no fundamental changes in the rhythm of the relationship that created the problems in the first place.

THE MANY FACES OF HER ANGER AND POWER DRIVES

Her repressed anger, rage, power, and control motives emerge in many indirect forms. Typically, the more femininely repressed she is, the more frequently these repressed responses occur and emerge as:

1. *Passive Aggression*—This occurs in the form of lateness, forgetting, procrastination, nonresponsiveness, untimely "accidents," misunderstanding, and undermining him by saying the wrong things in front of people and embarrassing him.
2. *Lack of Energy*—She's exhausted most of the time.

3. *Psychosomatic Complaints*—She has an ever-changing, endless, and exotic catalogue of physical illnesses and symptoms.
4. *Religious Fanaticism, Mysticism, and Moral Righteousness*—This is a potent form of gaining power indirectly.
5. *Complaining and Nagging*
6. *Crying, Blaming, and Other Emotional Displays of Pain and Hurt Designed to Make Him Feel Guilty*
7. *Emotional Breakdowns*
8. *Helplessness and Fear*
9. *Compulsive Homemaking and Mothering That Irritate Him*—These are a form of protesting too much on her part about her dedication to her role.

THE MANY FACES OF HIS RAGE

He has been taught to be protective and therefore has a ready tendency to feel guilty and responsible when things go wrong in an intimate relationship. This, plus a deep dependency on his woman and fear of loss of his sole "close" or "intimate" relationship, causes him to repress overt manifestations of his hostile or negative feelings. They too, therefore, take many passive and indirect forms. These include:

1. *Withdrawal and Nonresponsiveness*—The angrier he feels, the colder and more detached he becomes. He stays glued to endless numbers of sporting events on television, he's always "working," or simply doesn't hear her, or won't talk with her.
2. *Paternalism*—He demeans and indirectly puts her down by treating her as if she were a naive, stupid child.
3. *Criticalness and Sarcastic Humor*
4. *Intellectualization*—He never really tells her what he feels. Instead, he makes speeches and intellectualizes issues.
5. *Passive Indifference*
6. *Insensitivity*—He does certain things repeatedly to hurt her, even though she's told him on many occasions how they make her feel.
7. *Workaholism*
8. *Self-Destructiveness and Impulsiveness*—He drinks too much, gambles, drives recklessly, and takes chances that threaten the security of his family.

A FORMULA FOR SPOUSE VIOLENCE*

Spouse violence is the product of an interaction or rhythm between two people who are intensely dependent on each other and yet feel trapped, frustrated, and disappointed with each other at the same time. Neither is able to leave the relationship, and yet neither really wants to stay or feels fulfilled or comfortable.

The inevitable feelings of resentment, despair over making things better, and the deeper sense of being blocked by the other person from growing and being real make the relationship volatile. In some instances, the rage and feelings of being trapped emerge directly as physical violence. More commonly, in more controlled and "civilized" relationships, the rage is expressed in the previously discussed indirect forms via coldness, passive and indirect aggression, compulsive rituals, psychosomatic and emotional disorders, and hurtful verbal encounters.

In all of these interactions, no one is to blame, but both are victims of their unconscious gender defenses and the consciousness of themselves and their relationship that these produce.

The ingredients that set the stage for the rage that does produce physical attack include:

- A traditional woman whose childlike dependence and feelings of helplessness propel her to crave reassurance, contact, and closeness in a relationship with a machinelike male whose tendency is toward isolation ("leave me alone") and who has minimal tolerance for emotional and personal interaction. A vicious circle is created as she demands more and he wants less. He pulls deeper into himself and walls himself off as she becomes more desperately insistent and demanding of contact in a childlike, persistent way. While she complains of rejection, he complains of being smothered.

- A traditional man and woman who are unable to fight fairly and resolve conflict. She expresses her growing anger in irritatingly passive and hidden ways such as nagging, flirting, and blaming, while he handles his anger by coldly withdrawing, criticizing, and attempting to control his partner even more by withholding whatever she needs.

- An *actor-reactor* interaction that is basically boring to both, though neither has other resources to effectively change things. They cling to each other at the same time that the hunger for excitement and aloneness with others in each of them grows. Mutual provocation expresses their unconscious wish to push away from their partner.

- A traditional man and woman who are drawn to each other out of defensive needs and insecurity and are regressively dependent on each other at the same time that there is a latent hunger for further individual growth. The partner is needed yet resented as an obstacle to freedom and personal development at the same time.

- A man and woman who resent critical aspects of each other (i.e., He says, "You're too dependent on me") but are threatened by any changes their partner might attempt to make to improve matters. They continually block each other's changes in spite of expressed dissatisfaction with the way things are, and it becomes a "no-exit," "no-hope" matter.

- A situation in which the same basic fights repeat themselves over and over again. The intensity of rage and frustration increases, however, because of the grinding-down impact of the repetitions. Both feel abused, maligned, and unheard.

- A man who has needs but is fearful and unable to ask for what he wants, and resents it when he is not being correctly divined; and a woman who has needs for power and autonomy, but feels unable to directly take it and blames her husband for "controlling" her. In this interaction, he feels as if he's getting nothing, while everything is being demanded; and she feels she is being controlled. Both blame the other for their own defensive limitations.

- The continuing polarization of machine-man and child-woman, which causes him to see her increasingly as irresponsible, irrational, and insatiably needy; and causes her to see him as withholding, insensitive, cold, and unreachable.

- A woman who knows what she doesn't like, but has difficulty defining what she wants. She therefore responds negativistically toward a man who in turn feels unduly responsible and guilty, and is therefore overly sensitive to her complaints of dissatisfaction.

- A relationship that begins on a tremendous romantic high, with expectations that cannot be maintained, and is therefore followed inevitably by disappointment and feelings of betrayal.

Any one of a number of triggers can send these couples, who are sitting on these painful feelings and conflicts, into a physical confrontation that temporarily releases the rage and produces the distance that neither are able to establish in healthy, open, and productive ways.

THE GROWING FEAR OF EACH OTHER

With each succeeding generation, the repressed and experienced rage between the sexes increases and intensifies and produces a self-protective, phobic orientation. The fear of getting close is at one and the same time the fear of being destroyed and the fear of one's own destructive feelings toward the opposite sex. Relationships, therefore, tend to become increasingly more superficial, temporary, exploitative, and unsatisfying between men and women whose primary energies are going toward defensive maneuvers or "narcissism." Few relationships seem to maintain themselves without various, massive, indirect ways of creating a safe distance. In the extreme, some men and women lose their capacity for heterosexual relationships and no longer relate to each other intimately at all.

Men and women have both been victims of this socialization process that has caused them to fear and hate each other. Neither means the other harm. Each seeks desperately to attach in ways that feel good and are satisfying, but because of the process that is unconsciously created by gender defensiveness, they continually and unknowingly frustrate, disappoint, and feel "trapped" by each other.

5. Alcohol and Family Violence

Rodney J. Shapiro, Ph.D.
Director
Family Therapy Program
Veterans Administration Medical Center
San Francisco, California

Five

INCREASING EVIDENCE POINTS TO A SIGNIFICANT ASSOCIATION of alcohol and many forms of violence (Gerson, 1978; Pernanen, 1976). A number of investigations demonstrate that alcoholics are more aggressive and impulsive and score significantly higher on measures of hostility than do nonalcoholics (Williams, 1976). It is hardly surprising, then, that drinking is commonly implicated in family violence. Wife battering is most likely to occur when husbands are intoxicated, with the most extreme physical abuse being suffered by women whose spouses are consistent drinkers (Melville, 1978; Pernanen, 1976; Rosenbaum & O'Leary, 1981; Walker, 1979). There is also reason to believe that a high proportion of child abusers are alcoholics (Hanson & Estes, 1977; Pernanen, 1976, p. 365). Data were collected by the author at a clinic* providing evaluation and treatment for families presenting a wide variety of problems (Shapiro, in press). Approximately 20% of these families reported significant incidents of violence (mainly spouse abuse), and excessive drinking occurred in over half of these cases.

Ironically, family violence and alcoholism share another common characteristic, in that both have been unduly neglected by clinicians. Alcoholics are regarded as poor prospects for psychotherapy because of their characteristic irresponsibility, evasiveness, and inability to tolerate frustration (Shapiro, 1977). Violent individuals, whether or not they are alcoholics, evoke considerable anxiety in clinicians. Countertransference

---

*Marriage & Family Clinic, Psychiatry Department, University of Rochester Medical School, Rochester, New York (Barnhill, 1980a; Shapiro, 1977, in press).

reactions of fear and anger may prevent or impede treatment (Lion & Pasternak, 1973). The therapist's negative attitudes toward drinking and violence attach to the families as well as to the individuals themselves, and thus countertransference is compounded when working with more than one family member. Therapeutic engagement is also rendered less likely by the considerable resistance these families have towards treatment.

The present study is an attempt to redress the clinical neglect of these problems. Drinking and violent behavior are considered in the context of family systems, with a view to increasing our understanding of these phenomena and generating effective methods of evaluation and treatment. The data and conclusions are confined to families in which the alcoholic/violent individual is an adult male (though other members of these families may also exhibit similar behaviors at times). This emphasis is congruent with the general literature, in that most studies of alcoholism have focused on adult males (Gomberg, 1976), and the serious acts of family violence are usually inflicted by men (Straus, 1980).

TRADITIONAL PERSPECTIVES

Traditional views of alcoholism and violence reflect confusion about the conceptualization of these problems. Alcoholism is widely viewed as a medical disorder and most institutional treatment settings operate on this premise. However, there are contradictions inherent in this view of alcoholism, some of which actually obstruct the chances of therapeutic change (Shapiro, 1977). One striking characteristic of alcoholics is their penchant for disavowing responsibility for their actions or for changing their behavior. Translating their drinking into a medical problem simply fosters this very defense. The disease model of alcoholism also implies that some chemical substance may be discovered that will be utilized to "cure" the drinking. This again may reinforce the alcoholic's inclination to take a passive-dependent position in treatment. Despite these complications the disease perspective holds sway because it is based on the undeniable rationale that, regardless of etiology, the excessive use of alcohol is injurious to health (National Council on Alcoholism, 1972).

The disease definition implies that answers to questions of etiology lie within the organism. There have been many efforts to identify biological and intrapsychic determinants of alcoholism, but definite conclusions still elude us. Proponents of psychotherapy naturally emphasize the importance of psychological determinants, and a substantial literature has accumulated on the personality characteristics of the heavy drinker. Although personality factors do seem to be significant in the development of alcoholism, there has been little success in designating the ''alcoholic personality'' as an identifiable diagnostic entity (Williams, 1976). Characteristic behavioral patterns reflect aggression, self-pity and low self-esteem, but these may be consequences of the development of a chronic drinking problem rather than denoting inherent personality characteristics (Williams, 1976). Chafetz and his associates (1970) have observed that chronic depression, masked by denial, is characteristic of many alcoholics, but this condition is associated with other disorders too, and again it is difficult to determine whether this is a precursor or a subsequent development.

The traditional treatment approach to alcoholism requires an immediate curtailment of drinking, with institutionalization and medication as the primary methods of control. Additional treatment invariably includes some form of individual and group psychotherapy. Whatever the bias of the particular therapist, the goal is to evoke changes in the individual patient that will result in future abstinence from alcohol. The effectiveness of traditional psychotherapy for alcoholism remains unsubstantiated (Chafetz et al. 1970, 1974), but these methods still prevail in most treatment settings.

The problem of violence resists definition as a disease process. The criterion of a noxious entity precipitating symptomatology does not apply to violence as it does to alcoholism. The expression of violence encompasses social, cultural, legal, and psychological factors. Psychiatric involvement has been limited to violence as an occasional aspect of psychopathology, or as a manifestation of neurological or physiological dysfunction. Violence is sometimes associated with a variety of acute psychiatric disturbances, and interventions emphasize management by means of physical restraint, seclusion, and tranquilizers. If disturbances of neurological, hormonal, and other biological functions are detected, corrective medications become the treatment of choice. In the absence of symptomatology, violence may be defined as a behavioral disorder such as delinquency or sociopathy. Whether individuals presenting such behavior should fit into the purview of psychiatry or the law remains a point of debate.

As noted earlier, clinicians are generally reluctant to work with violent individuals in psychotherapy. However, such contact is sometimes unavoidable. The therapist who sees alcoholics is inevitably confronted with, or learns about, acts of violence. The commonly observed association of drinking and violence is traditionally explained as a cause-effect sequence. It is assumed that alcohol "causes" violence, and this viewpoint dominates most research on the subject as well as treatment methodology. This "direct cause" explanation is a compaction of the widely accepted "disinhibition theory" of alcohol use, namely that alcohol reduces the inhibition of aggressive impulses (Pernanen, 1976).

Therapists who subscribe to this theory work with the expectation that the violence will cease when the alcoholic gives up drinking. Such reasoning stems from traditional conceptualizations of individual psychopathology that are based on linear sequences of cause and effect. In this instance the sequence would be that early life experiences lead to the development of particular personality characteristics. These predispose the individual to heavy drinking. The excessive intake of alcohol weakens the inhibition of impulses, including aggression. Psychotherapy may emphasize self-awareness so that an understanding of early experiences and (overt and covert) personality functioning will free the individual from reliance on alcohol and inability to control his or her violent urges.

AN INTERACTIONAL PERSPECTIVE

Traditional treatment approaches have focused on understanding and changing the individual who is alcoholic and violent. In recent years there have been attempts to broaden this perspective by placing less emphasis on intrapsychic causation and giving more recognition to interpersonal determinants of behavior. In the field of alcohol research this trend has been reflected in the growing awareness that families are somehow implicated in the problems of the individual alcoholic. An early step in this direction can be seen in studies of alcoholic spouses. It has long been suspected that wives of alcoholics suffer personality disturbances such that they tend to select alcoholic mates to satisfy unconscious needs. The clinical relevance of this supposition is that these women tend to undermine their husbands' attempts to control drinking. Research data, however, have not identified a unitary personality type for the wives of alcoholics. These findings have been summarized by Ablon (1976) and Jacob and his colleagues (1978).

The limiting factor in these studies is similar to that in research on the alcoholic personality: there is an underlying assumption that certain personality variables "cause" specific behaviors. Understanding family members in addition to the alcoholic is a necessary but insufficient step in the right direction. It is the relationship between family members that provides the key element for an enhanced understanding of such problems as drinking and violence.

The interactional model stems in large part from the influence of systems theory (Bertalanffy, 1966) and the development of family therapy (Guerin, 1976). A radical and far-reaching new perspective on alcoholism has resulted from the introduction of family theory. The central premise of this viewpoint is that drinking may have adaptive consequences in maintaining stability of family relationships (Chafetz et al. 1974; Davis, Berenson, Steinglass, & Davis, 1974). Recent studies of alcoholic-spouse interaction are adding considerably to our understanding of alcoholism, and suggest that treatment be focused on family relationships rather than on individuals (Gorad, 1971; Gorad, McCourt, & Cobb, 1971; Kennedy, 1976).

Family theory has only recently begun to impact on studies of family violence. There have been increasing signs of dissatisfaction with traditional intrapsychic theories of violence (Pernanen, 1976; Shapiro, in press). The expression of violence always occurs in a context of complex interactions. Variables such as marital conflict, alcohol intake, and violence are not linked in a linear sequence of cause-effect, but impinge on each other in circular fashion so that no one factor is "cause" or "effect." For example, marital conflict may be a reaction to drinking, which in turn leads to increased drinking, which exacerbates conflict leading to violence, and so on. Violent behavior is complex and cannot simply be defined as one individual gratuitously inflicting abuse on another. Family violence must be understood as a component of interactions between family members (Shapiro, in press).

Earlier, we considered the "direct cause" theory of alcohol-related violence. We are now in a position to better understand the limitations of this viewpoint. Alcohol cannot "cause" violence; it can only reduce inhibitions so that violence is more likely to be expressed in the context of a particular set of interactions. Studies of alcohol-related spouse abuse already provide clear evidence that alcohol is a catalyst rather than a cause of violence (Martin, 1978; Melville, 1978; Walker, 1979). Anger and hostility are generated by interactions between couples (and other family members), not by the intake of alcohol.

Conceptualizing alcoholism and violence in terms of family theory provides a comprehensive explanatory model, and appears to offer the most favorable prospects for amelioration of these problems (Davis et al. 1974; Shapiro, 1977, in press). This perspective has the added advantage of resolving the contradictions inherent in the view of the offender as "sick" and therefore not responsible for his or her behavior, and it also counters the tendency for families (and therapists) to blame the violent or alcoholic individual for whatever difficulties exist in the family.

CLINICAL CONSIDERATIONS

If we view both violence and drinking disorders as interactional behaviors, it stands to reason that we need firsthand knowledge of the social context in which these behaviors occur. In practice, this requires the participation of the whole family unit in the evaluation phase and if necessary in the actual treatment process as well. When marital discord is the presenting problem it may be expedient to see the couple first and include the children later. In cases of child abuse or parent abuse it is advisable to involve all members of the household at an early stage of the evaluation. Family therapists are well aware of the complexities involved in engaging families when one member is clearly designated as the index patient. Techniques for initially involving family members are employed by all family therapists and these will not be elaborated here. The interested reader may refer to several helpful articles in a recent collection of clinical issues by Gurman (1981). Characteristic patterns of resistance emerge once contact is actually established with violent and alcoholic families, and these will be considered in the context of evaluation and treatment.

The Evaluation Phase

Most clinical and research studies on drinking and violence relate to families or individuals that come to appropriate treatment agencies for help with these difficulties. However, there are families or individuals who seek treatment for any number of other reasons, and only at some point after the initial contact is it learned that there may be drinking or violence involved. Whether these problems are initially presented or they emerge later reflects two significantly different clinical situations. The family that presents with these difficulties is at least not resistant to admitting their existence. The therapist does not have to struggle to bring the problems out into the open. However, the family that resists revealing these problems has strong reasons for believing that they should be kept secret. Family loyalty or fears of retribution may be involved. In these cases, the task of the therapist is to facilitate the full disclosure of such difficulties. Guarantees against retribution may be necessary, particularly for children. Families may differ in admitting to either drinking or violence, depending on which activity is considered less defensible.

The identity of the members involved in drinking and violence must be ascertained rather than inferred. Families may include several drinkers and abusive persons, but for various reasons identify only one as the index patient. Wives are known to be as frequently assaultive as husbands (Straus, 1980), but they are less likely to be defined as violent because their attacks seldom result in physical damage. A large-scale study of marital violence revealed that in approximately half of the assaultive incidents both spouses had been drinking (Gerson, 1978). The identification of offenders and victims may expose situations of spouse abuse, child abuse, or parent abuse, and enable the clinician to formulate appropriate interventions (Shapiro, in press).

An early determination should be made as to the severity and current phase of both drinking and violence. An accurate estimate will influence treatment strategy and bear on prognosis. Clinicians should not rely on subjective statements. One family member or another may report that the drinking ''is not a big problem,'' but when the facts are obtained a very different picture may emerge. Information about the extent of alcoholic intake must be considered in relation to the current phase of drinking. If this is a family in which an individual has only recently begun drinking, we have a very different situation from a family in which one member has a long-term drinking habit. The beginning drinker, particularly if the intake is not very heavy, is more likely to deny the seriousness of his or her problem. In this case, though, the family is not yet accustomed to this behavior and may be more accessible to change. On the other hand, the chronic alcoholic and his or her family may readily admit to the drinking but prove extremely resistant to therapeutic change. Determining the extent and current status of violent behavior is equally important. There is a major difference between the family with a history of occasional violence and one in which violence occurs regularly. Again, the chronicity of the problem relates to resistance. The family with occasional violence is more likely to experience it as dystonic and may be more motivated to change the situation. The family that has tolerated violence for many years may be less likely to accept the changes necessary to end the abuse.

A family evaluation must include a diagnostic assessment of each individual, particularly the violent alcoholic. Factors that exacerbate violence may involve neurological dysfunction (Elliott, 1976) and abuse of substances other than alcohol (Roy, 1977). A pathological reaction to alcohol is rare, but may account for the sudden eruption of rage in an individual without a prior history of violence (Banay, 1944; Cohen, 1981). Some sources of influence are not evident in the clinical setting, but may be significant. These include financial and occupational stresses and cultural attitudes toward drinking and violence (Lystad, 1975; Straus, 1977).

The main thrust of the evaluation is classification of the family's characteristic style of functioning. Communication patterns (verbal and nonverbal) reveal the matrix of relationships and clarify the function that symptoms and behaviors serve in the family system. The interactional sequences in these families, particularly between the marital partners, tend to foster the drinking and violent behaviors (Bullock & Mudd, 1959; Mitchell, 1959; Shapiro, in press). This issue will be considered again in the section on treatment.

Crisis Intervention

In cases in which a family is at a crisis point and both drinking and violence are problems, then immediate interventions may be necessary. The individual who is in the midst of a drinking bout is typically not capable of engaging in an extended evaluation or meaningful therapy, and may actually have to be institutionalized for a period of time to "dry out." Likewise, direct interventions may be called for if a family is currently experiencing violence. This may include separation of the offender and victims, and possible institutionalization in the event of uncontrolled drinking or an acute psychotic episode. Principles of family crisis intervention were enunciated by Langsley and his co-workers (1968), and a useful guide to crisis intervention for cases of intrafamilial violence has been provided by Barnhill (1980b).

A question that may arise during the evaluation is whether to give priority to the drinking or to the violence, should both occur in the same family. There is no general answer to this question since it would very much depend on the particular family, and the impact of these behaviors on the system. However, some guidelines can be suggested. When violence is occurring or threatening to occur, then immediate attention has to be given to this problem. The drinking should be acknowledged as something that has to be dealt with, but the first priority is to stop the violence. In order to do this (barring institutionalization or physical separation) the therapist can provide a rule that forbids violence. In the clinic in Rochester we had considerable success in formulating rules forbidding violence when working with families (Shapiro, in press). The rules are most effective once the family is involved in treatment, but may work well even if advocated during an initial contact. Generally, both the perpetrator and victim are unhappy with the situation and prefer not to have violent confrontations or enforced separation. However, these individuals are not capable of changing the situation themselves. The violent individual, by the very nature of the problem, is unable to contain himself or herself at a certain point in the interaction with the victim. On the other hand, the victim does not have the power to stop the violent behavior either. Should the victim attempt to establish a rule forbidding violence, the antagonist is likely to perceive it as a threat and this could trigger another abusive response. Only the therapist has the neutrality and power to impose the rule and this seems to work well. What seems to work best, from our own experience, is to agree with the family that one of the partners involved will leave the home should the violent episode occur and spend a designated period of time away from the other. This rule is extremely effective for two reasons. First, it allows either partner to literally take distance, a maneuver that invariably helps to prevent or impede violence, and second, separation is an especially significant consequence since it is experienced as particularly distressing to these families. If the situation entails a high probability of further violence, then legal interventions, or recourse to refuges for battered women, or other immediate means of separation may be necessary.

In those families in which violence is not viewed as serious but somewhat syntonic, and is not currently a crisis issue, the drinking may need to be given priority. If an individual is alcoholic and while intoxicated becomes violent, then the therapist has to confront the family with the requirement that the drinking cease immediately in order to deal with the violence and other problems. Alcoholism is unlikely to be curtailed solely on the basis of outpatient contacts. Initially, the alcoholic may require a controlled period of mandatory abstinence in an appropriate treatment facility. The family should be involved as part of the treatment from the outset. Particularly important will be the family's involvement in treatment following discharge. It is a common experience for alcoholics to dry out in a matter of several weeks in a treatment facility and then shortly after discharge resume their drinking.

General Treatment Principles

Within the field of family therapy there are strongly divergent practices, and there is no reason to suppose that one method is most successful in treating families with drinking problems and violence. In formulating the dynamics of each case I rely on psychodynamic concepts as well as family systems theory (Shapiro, 1980). Interventions based on structural family therapy (Minuchin, 1974) have proven effective, particularly when parent-child problems are salient. Techniques derived from strategic family therapy (Madanes, 1981) and paradoxical methods inspired by the Palazzoli group (1978) have been employed successfully with inflexible and resistant families.

The central issue in working with these families is that of resistance. At the outset, the clinician must begin to unravel the covert resistance behind the expressed desire for change. Different aspects of resistance may emerge during the course of the treatment process. Each individual may have reason to perceive therapy as threatening and accordingly resorts to a characteristic defensive style. The most critical task for the therapist is to clarify recurring interactional patterns since those that most resist change are also likely to contribute to the drinking and abusive behavior.

Structuring the Treatment

Families with drinking and violence as problems have difficulty in accepting the structure and expectations inherent in traditional psychotherapy. Such families have members that are often unreliable, unable to tolerate the slow pace of insight-oriented therapy, and strongly inclined to manipulate the therapist. A characteristic style of interaction for these families is that of sidetaking and blaming, and they attempt to set up the therapist as a referee (Shapiro, 1977). When tensions rise during sessions there is an increased risk of subsequent drinking or violence. For these reasons it is imperative that the therapist assume a strong and consistent posture from the first contact with the family, even from the first telephone contact.

The therapist needs to control the process of treatment, set rules, and stick to them. Some of these rules relate to the customary conditions of therapy, such as duration and frequency of sessions, fees, membership requirements at sessions, and so on. The most significant rules pertain to the curtailment of violence and drinking. It is generally easier to control the violence than the drinking. Families seldom resort to physical assaults during sessions, particularly if such behavior is expressly forbidden by the therapist. Furthermore, as noted earlier, the collaborative setting of rules against violence at home is usually effective once treatment gets underway. Sobriety is much more difficult to enforce. Although the therapist can set rules against intoxication during sessions, it is almost impossible to control alcohol abuse outside of the therapeutic hour. From my experience with many such families, I have come to the conclusion that it is unrealistic to demand total abstinence if working only on an outpatient basis. Heavy drinkers usually require some period of institutional control in order to begin an attempt at total abstinence.

Case Example

A couple presented with an unusual problem of violence. The wife would sometimes be awakened during the night as her husband was hitting her and attempting to choke her. He claimed to be in a ''sleep state'' during these episodes, and they always followed an evening of heavy drinking. Curiously, the wife did not complain about her husband's drinking, but only about these episodic night attacks.

The interactional pattern between this couple was striking for its mutual blaming, and competitiveness. Each bemoaned a lack of emotional support and respect from the other. The couple was unable to focus for any length of time on a specific issue, tended to escalate conflicts by assailing each other with accusations of numerous past offenses, and rarely attempted to resolve problems. It was learned that various attempts at treatment in the past had been unsuccessful.

Much of the therapy emphasized rules and limitsetting, both for the treatment process as well as the couple's interaction. Initially, the husband challenged the therapist's authority by bringing liquor to the sessions, arriving intoxicated, and talking in a loud and aggressive manner. The therapist, who was still in training, felt intimidated, but with supervisory support he assumed control. The husband gradually tolerated and accepted rules about no liquor or intoxication during sessions. The violence ceased but the drinking at home increased. The therapist confronted the couple with the necessity for an inpatient alcohol program in conjunction with marital therapy. The husband agreed but kept procrastinating. The wife was unenthusiastic and less interested in therapy now that the violence had subsided. After a period of sporadic attendance the couple decided to stop treatment, but left a message declaring their intention of resuming again in the future.

Sources of Resistance

Families with problems of alcohol or violence tend to seek help at a time of crisis. At that point there appears to be strong motivation for treatment. Remarkably, though, once the crisis has passed, these families seem reluctant to continue in therapy.

A careful exploration of the motivations for contacting our clinic revealed that while complaints about drinking and violence were frequently presented, the precipitants for seeking treatment were usually related to an actual or threatened separation. A typical scenario would precede the request for treatment. A family conflict arose at a time when the husband was intoxicated. It escalated to the point of violence and the wife threatened to leave. Such threats were frequent, but this time the wife seemed determined. The husband attempted to appease her. He swore that he did not want to strike her and would never do it again. She remained unmoved and reminded him of previous broken promises. He reiterated that he would never strike her again and declared his intention of giving up alcohol. She demanded that he get professional help. He agreed.

Some such negotiation is the impetus for many couples who seek help. As long as the wife's threat has force, the husband will ''behave himself'' by trying not to drink and by restraining his violence and attending therapy sessions. After a period of time the crisis usually fades, the resistance of the husband becomes apparent, and the wife, who is equally resistant, makes only weak attempts to persuade the husband to continue in treatment. Once again the wife can postpone the separation issue and avoid therapy by blaming the husband for his resistance or the therapist for being ineffective. The husband has fulfilled his promise to seek treatment, and he can deny his resistance but agree with his wife that the therapy was not effective.

It is generally acknowledged that alcoholics, like other addicts, have great difficulty in conquering their habit. What is less widely known, and far less credible, is that the spouses of alcoholics are also resistant to changes that might bring about termination of the drinking (Chafetz et al. 1974; Meeks & Kelly, 1970). An explanation for the resistance of the spouse lies in the suggestion that the drinking serves a purpose in stabilizing the interactional functioning of the family system (Chafetz et al. 1974; Davis et al.1974).

Thus, fear of separation seems to be a core marital issue in these families (Shapiro, 1977). When conflict and distress are greatest either spouse may consider separation, but the idea seldom achieves resolution. Therapy may be threatening because of a not unrealistic fear that honest confrontations might lead to separation. The wife who faces the fact that she cannot change her husband has to either accept the situation or give up on the marriage. The husband who gives up drinking may no longer need the qualities of his wife that were once important to him.

Case Example

A man of 57 and his 39-year-old wife sought treatment following a suicide attempt by the husband. The precipitant was the wife's decision to separate. She moved out of the house after a fierce argument over finances had culminated in her being struck by the husband. After she left he attempted suicide and was hospitalized. The wife promised to return and did so when he was discharged.

Both partners had been previously married and had grown-up children. The current union had lasted seven years, during which time the husband had struck his wife on three occasions. In recalling how they met the husband remembered being drawn to her youthful vivacity, her admiration of him, and her sympathetic concern. She had been attracted to his warm, fatherly qualities, and was impressed by his mysterious and exciting business ventures. He had a history of alcohol abuse, but she was a qualified nurse and believed she could help him with this problem. As time passed the wife's admiration waned. She realized that his secret business practices were questionable and generally unsuccessful, and that he was unsupportive and increasingly dependent and demanding. He felt that her initial concern was replaced by an unsympathetic bossiness.

The most intense conflicts centered on money. The husband was in constant financial difficulty, and he rejected the wife's inquiries and advice as denoting a lack of confidence and disrespect. She felt insecure about their financial situation, felt compelled to question him, and felt demeaned by his rejection of her offers of assistance.

This pattern of interaction was reflected in all areas of disagreement. Seemingly trivial issues would trigger heated arguments. One such incident might well have led to violence if the couple had not been in therapy at the time. The wife had complained about a malfunctioning appliance and the husband related the problem to faulty wiring in the house. He devoted himself to a complicated and time-consuming modification of the wiring. The wife protested that he was unqualified to undertake such a project, and that it was probably unnecessary anyway. She felt endangered by the risk that defective work could result in fire or electrocution. The husband was enraged that his efforts were unappreciated and his skills unrecognized. She was infuriated by his refusal to heed her concerns and objections.

Such intense struggles were frequent. When a stalemate was reached the wife might resort to her "trump card," which was a threat to quit the marriage. The husband would back down or counter with threats or actual violence. They would often avert a showdown by seeking out allies or a referee. This maneuver carried into treatment. They put great pressure on the therapist to take sides, and it was only with difficulty that they learned to listen to each other and actually begin to collaborate rather than fight. The violence disappeared immediately after the commencement of therapy, and this couple made steady but slow progress towards achieving a more amicable relationship.

Creating Therapeutic Alliances

If resistance is a primary issue in the treatment of these families, then it stands to reason that the therapist should recognize and work with such resistance from the start. Therapy is more likely to continue beyond the initial crisis if the therapist can succeed in forming a strong alliance with key members of the family. Where marital discord is the primary issue, the therapist must aim at developing an alliance with the husband and wife. Where children are involved, particularly in cases of child abuse or parent abuse, the affected child and siblings must also be positively engaged by the therapist.

Alcoholics and their mates often have defensive styles that hamper the clinician's efforts to establish a therapeutic alliance (Shapiro, 1977). The alcoholic, whether or not he or she is violent, tends to be extremely defensive, self-centered, and hypersensitive to criticism. He or she feels like a failure and may indulge in self-recrimination and vows of good intentions, but more often than not these declarations represent elaborate avoidance rather than spurs to action. The therapist has to maintain a nonjudgmental stance, offer patient support, and resist personal disappointment or anger in the face of inevitable setbacks.

Establishing a positive working alliance with the spouse is problematic but absolutely essential. For many wives of alcoholics the therapist represents both a source of help and a threat. They look to the therapist for understanding and some alleviation of the considerable stress they experience. More often than not the wife has shouldered the burden of raising the children, taking charge of the household, and working to ensure a consistent income. In relation to her husband she typically assumes the role of caretaker and manager. She holds to the view that the husband is the only disturbed family member, and that all their problems are due to his drinking. She resists experiencing herself as the patient. Needless to say, the alcoholic's spouse poses a formidable challenge to the therapist. The therapist meets resistance when shifting the exploratory focus from the husband to her. She may contend with the therapist in determining the direction of sessions, and she may collude with the husband in neutralizing clinical input that threatens change.

Inexperienced therapists have particular difficulty with these women. Power struggles between therapist and wife are common, and center on who decides the content and process of sessions. The most effective posture for the therapist is to join with rather than struggle against the wife. The empathic appreciation of her hardships is appropriate and likely to win her cooperation. Instead of vying for control, the therapist should acknowledge the wife's "expertise." Providing empathy, support, and validation ironically gives the therapist considerable power and control without being controlling. If the therapist is not threatened and competitive (unlike the husband), the wife can shed her armor and become receptive to therapy for herself.

The role of the children in these families is frequently overlooked to the detriment of treatment. When drinking is a chronic problem the role of the alcoholic parent may be shared by the other spouse and one parentified child. That child has a partial stake in maintaining the family system in order to preserve his or her role, and this source of resistance can be significant. The therapist should work closely with the parentified child, and involve the other siblings as well.

Restoring the alcoholic parent to a fully functioning role in the family is no easy matter. When problems have persisted for many years, the typical structure in these families is that of a wife with her children forming one boundaried unit with the offending spouse as a relative outsider. Attempts on his part to enter the system, for example by exerting discipline or achieving intimacy with the wife, meet with such resistance that he is likely to resort to drinking again or to violence. On the other hand, should the wife and children provide an opportunity for the husband to function more fully, his own ambivalence is likely to ensure failure and consequently reinforce his exclusion from the rest of the family. The therapist can counter this reciprocal resistance by making the interactional sequences explicit, and acknowledging the difficulties for all concerned in attempting to change the structure of the family.

A particularly difficult problem for the family therapist is created by the countertransference reactions that are inevitable in working with violence. This problem has been amplified in greater detail elsewhere (Shapiro, in press). It is virtually impossible for the therapist to maintain objectivity and neutrality in the face of violent behavior. It is typical and understandable that the initial attitude toward the perpetrator is one of dislike, fear, or aversion, while the victim is generally regarded with sympathy. As we saw in our own work, though, these reactions tend to change over time. During treatment, the therapist invariably discovers the wife's hostility as well. Negative countertransference reactions then tend to shift from the husband to the wife. With continued contact these shifts tend to stabilize as the therapist gains understanding of the relationship as one in which there is mutual anger and hostility.

Countertransference reactions are particularly intense in cases of child abuse. The child abuser, whether or not he or she is alcoholic, rarely elicits warmth or sympathy in others. The challenge for the therapist is to involve that individual in treatment despite strong negative feelings. Working with the whole family is the most likely method for avoiding the trap of casting one family member in an extremely negative light. In our experience we found that even the child abuser could be viewed with some neutrality or even positive understanding once his or her role in the family system became understandable. An important dimension in this regard is the experience of the abuser in his or her own family of origin. Many violent adults have suffered abuse as children. Understanding their past experiences can lessen the temptation to fix blame.

CONCLUSIONS

Drinking and violence are pervasive problems in American family life, yet until recently there has been little clinical concern with these areas.

Family therapists are now beginning to reconsider these problems as interactional phenomena, and attempts to utilize family therapy as a mode of intervention for working with these problems seem to hold promise. However, a number of practical and theoretical questions need to be addressed in future studies.

With problems of such severity treatment is seldom restricted to one form of intervention. Utilizing an inpatient facility may be necessary (particularly for alcoholism), and the index patient will be involved in whatever treatment interventions prevail at that unit. Outpatient treatment also incorporates different methods, including medication, and individual and group therapy. The problem is how best to implement family therapy in a varied treatment milieu. Derivative questions would relate to which treatment modality should have priority, and how to resolve the contradictions of deemphasizing one family member as the patient when the overall treatment context is based on the identification of that individual as the patient.

The relationship of alcoholism and violence also needs further clarification. As we have seen, there is considerable confusion with regard to the question of cause and effect in understanding the association of alcohol and violence. Many factors are involved in problems as complex as these. It would be overly reductionistic to explain these phenomena purely in terms of family interaction. We already know that aggression is related to biological and psychological aspects of individual functioning, and that social and cultural factors influence these behaviors. A true systems approach for a full understanding of violence and drinking should incorporate all relevant variables, but it will take considerable time and effort to achieve this goal. At this juncture, the family therapy approach represents a significant advance in clinical understanding and provides methods of intervention that enhance the effectiveness of psychotherapy.

REFERENCES

Ablon, J. Family structure and behavior in alcoholism: A review of the literature. In B. Kissin & H. Begleiter (Eds.),*The biology of alcoholism, Vol. 4: Social aspects of alcoholism.* New York: Plenum Press, 1976.

Banay, R.S. Pathological reaction to alcohol. *Quarterly Journal of Studies on Alcohol*, 1944, *4*, 580–604.

Barnhill, L.R. Clinical assessment of intrafamilial violence. *Hospital and Community Psychiatry*, 1980, *31*, 543–546. (a)

Barnhill, L.R. Basic interventions for violence in families. *Hospital and Community Psychiatry*, 1980, *31*, 547–551. (b)

Bertalanffy, L. General system theory and psychiatry. In S. Arieti (Ed.), *American handbook of psychiatry, Vol. 3*. New York: Basic Books, 1966.

Bullock, S.C., & Mudd, E.H. The interaction of alcoholic husbands and their nonalcoholic wives during counseling. *American Journal of Orthopsychiatry*, 1959, *29*, 519–527.

Chafetz, M.E., Blane, H.T., & Hill, M.J. (Eds.). *Frontiers of alcoholism*. New York: Science House, 1970.

Chafetz, M.E., Hertzman, J., & Berenson, D. Alcoholism: A positive view. In S. Arieti & E.B. Brody (Eds.), *American handbook of psychiatry, Vol. 3, 2nd ed.* New York: Basic Books, 1974.

Cohen, S. Pathological intoxication. *Drug Abuse & Alcoholism Newsletter*, 1981, *10* (5).

Davis, D.I., Berenson, D., Steinglass, P., & Davis S. The adaptive consequences of drinking. *Psychiatry*, 1974, *37*, 209–215.

Elliott, F.A. Neurological factors in violent behavior (The dyscontrol syndrome). *Bulletin of the American Academy of Psychiatry and Law*, 1976, *4*, 297–315.

Gerson, L.W. Alcohol-related acts of violence: Who was drinking and where the acts occurred. *Journal of Studies on Alcohol*, 1978, *39*, 1294–1296.

Gomberg, E.S. Alcoholism in women. In B. Kissin & H. Begleiter (Eds.), *The biology of alcoholism, Vol. 4: Social aspects of alcoholism*. New York: Plenum Press, 1976.

Gorad, S.L. Communication styles and interaction of alcoholics and their wives. *Family Process*, 1971, *10*, 475–489.

Gorad, S.L., McCourt, W.S., & Cobb, J.C. A communications approach to alcoholism. *Quarterly Journal of Studies on Alcohol*, 1971, *32*, 651–668.

Guerin, P.J. Family therapy: The first twenty-five years. In P.J. Guerin (Ed.), *Family therapy: Theory and practice*. New York: Gardner Press, 1976.

Gurman, A.S. (Ed.). *Questions and answers in the practice of family therapy*. New York: Brunner/Mazel, 1981.

Hanson, K.J., & Estes, N.J. Dynamics of alcoholic families. In N.J. Estes & M.E. Heinemann (Eds.), *Alcoholism: Development, consequences, and interventions*. Saint Louis: C.V. Mosby, 1977.

Jacob, T., Favorini, A., Meisel, S.S., & Anderson, C.M. The alcoholic's spouse children and family interactions. *Journal of Studies on Alcohol*, 1978, *39*, 1231–1251.

Kennedy, D.L. Behavior of alcoholics and spouses in a simulation game situation. *Journal of Nervous and Mental Disease*, 1976, *162*, 23–34.

Langsley, D.G., Kaplan, D., Pittman, F., Machotka, P., Flomenhaft, K., & DeYoung, C. *The treatment of families in crisis*. New York: Grune & Stratton, 1968.

Lion, J.R., & Pasternak, S.A. Countertransference reactions to violent patients. *American Journal of Psychiatry*, 1973, *130*, 207–210.

Lystad, M.H. Violence at home: A review of the literature. *American Journal of Orthopsychiatry*, 1975, *45*, 328–345.

Madanes, C. *Strategic family therapy*. San Francisco: Jossey-Bass, 1981.

Martin, J.P. Some reflections on violence and the family. In J.P. Martin (Ed.), *Violence and the family*. New York: Wiley, 1978.

Meeks, D.E., & Kelly, C. Family therapy with the families of recovering alcoholics. *Quarterly Journal of Studies on Alcohol*, 1970, *31*, 399–413.

Melville, J. Women in refuges. In J.P. Martin (Ed.), *Violence and the family*. New York: Wiley, 1978.

Minuchin, S. *Families and family therapy.* Cambridge, Mass.: Harvard University Press, 1974.

Mitchell, H.E. Interpersonal perception theory applied to conflicted marriages in which alcoholism is and is not a problem. *American Journal of Orthopsychiatry,* 1959, *29,* 547–559.

National Council on Alcoholism. Criteria for the diagnosis of alcoholism. *American Journal of Psychiatry,* 1972, *129,* 127–135.

Palazzoli, M.S., Cecchin, E., Prata, G., & Boscolo, L. *Paradox and counterparadox.* New York: Jason Aronson, 1978.

Pernanen, K. Alcohol and crimes of violence. In B. Kissin & H. Begleiter (Eds.), *The biology of alcoholism, Vol. 4: Social aspects of alcoholism.* New York: Plenum Press, 1976.

Rosenbaum, A., & O'Leary, K.D. Marital violence: Characteristics of abusive couples. *Journal of Consulting and Clinical Psychology,* 1981, *49,* 63–71.

Roy, M. (Ed.) *Battered women: A psychosociological study of domestic violence.* New York: Van Nostrand Reinhold, 1977.

Shapiro, R.J. A family therapy approach to alcoholism. *Journal of Marriage and Family Counseling,* 1977, *3,* 71–78.

Shapiro, R.J. Psychodynamically oriented family therapy. In G.P. Sholevar, R.M. Benson, & B.J. Blinder (Eds.), *Emotional disorders in children and adolescents.* New York: Spectrum, 1980.

Shapiro, R.J. Therapy with violent families. In A. Anderson, C. Hart, & J. Rubenstein (Eds.), *Violent individuals and families: A practitioners' handbook.* Springfield, Ill.: Charles C Thomas, in press.

Straus, M. A sociological perspective on the prevention and treatment of wife beating. In M. Roy (Ed.), *Battered women: A psychosociological study of domestic violence.* New York: Van Nostrand Reinhold, 1977.

Straus, M. Victims and aggressors in marital violence. *American Behavioral Scientist,* 1980, *23,* 681–704.

Walker, L.E. *The battered woman,* New York: Harper & Row, 1979.

Williams, A.F. The alcoholic personality. In B. Kissin & H. Begleiter (Eds.), *The biology of alcoholism, Vol. 4: Social aspects of alcoholism.* New York: Plenum Press, 1976.

6. Adolescent Violence in the Family

Denis J. Madden, Ph.D.
Director, Clinical Research Program for
  Violent Behavior
Assistant Professor
Department of Psychiatry
University of Maryland School of Medicine
Baltimore, Maryland

Six

MURDER IS THE MOST EXTREME FORM OF ADOLESCENT violence. The lives of 10 youngsters, all below the age of 18, who murdered or attempted murder, are examined in Muriel Gardiner's book *The Deadly Innocents* (1976). Gardiner attempts to understand these youngsters by exploring the confluence of such variables as the perpetrators—themselves victims of life **forces**—a suitable victim, an outburst of rage, and the time and place to express that rage. These youngsters, she insists, are ''real people.''

Whenever we deal with a violent individual, we must constantly remind ourselves that, despite the seemingly inhuman behavior, the violent person is a ''real'' individual. The real horror lies not in the individual but in the deed and, even more so, in the fact that the deed need not have happened.

All violent crime leaves us questioning how such things could happen; how could one human being act so brutally against another person? Newspaper accounts and news reports on television may satisfy the popular need to be informed and to be stimulated by the sensational. Those in the mental health profession and other serious-minded persons find themselves driven to achieve a deeper understanding that might help stem the flow of violent crime. This paper works toward that purpose in presenting dynamics observed from contact with violent adolescents and their families. Statistical surveys on rates of crime are not presented, nor is an attempt made to review the delinquency literature. Mention is made of those family interactional studies that lead to a fuller understanding of family dynamics.

MYTHS

Visceral issues like violence can lead to prejudice, and prejudice can lead to the establishment of myths. Several myths that surround discussions of violent adolescents are challenged by a recent study of Hamparian and her colleagues (1978). What she discovered among Columbus, Ohio, youths was that juvenile violent offenders constituted a very small fraction of the total number of youths in that city. These juveniles did not typically progress from less serious to more serious crimes. Status offenders (adolescents who violate curfews, are truant, or are run-aways) did not appear to be headed toward a confirmed criminal career. And, not surprisingly, institutional commitment does not prevent delinquency or rehabilitate the violent offender.

Another myth is that adolescent violence is an American phenomenon or a product of the West. A recent report in the *Washington Post* (1982) cites several brutal violent crimes committed by adolescents in Russia. In one account an adolescent named Kotov killed his mother because she was a heavy drinker. As the *Post* reports, "Although the murder was described in a series of two articles, the reasons for Kotov's action remain obscure." There is always much that remains obscure when dealing with the issue of violence. Part of the reason for this is that we are dealing with real people and real people are quite complex—especially during the adolescent period.

There is a general lack of understanding of what motivates people to commit violent crimes. Despite this fact, clinicians are called upon to offer guidance in dealing with the phenomenon of human aggression. One is challenged from the outset with the question of who is the patient and who is in need of treatment—the adolescent, the family, or society. Violence cannot be isolated, nor can those who commit violent crimes be isolated or singled out as the sole perpetrators of violent crimes. The lack of impulse control on the part of adolescents who engage in violent behavior makes them the most likely candidates for becoming the identified patients.

FAMILY DYNAMICS

One way to better understand adolescent violence is to be aware of family dynamics and the interaction of family members. Clinical case reports of children and adolescents who have committed violent acts give some insight into the family dynamics, along with individual pathological correlates and even the possible neurological concomitants of violent adolescents.

The homes of adolescents who are violent are described as being quite chaotic in their organization. At times the parents are overly punitive and restrictive, and at other times approving of and encouraging the use of violence by the adolescents (Duncan & Duncan, 1971; Scherl & Mack, 1966; King, 1975; Easson & Steinhilber, 1961; Sadoff, 1971; Kalogerakis, 1972). In fact, one study states "that only where there is parental permission is the child's conflict acted out in lethal violence" (Easson & Steinhilber, 1961). It also has been hypothesized that adolescent aggressiveness may well be an acting out of parental antisocial impulses. Thus, violent behavior is dealt with inconsistently, sometimes punished and sometimes rewarded.

Parental ties with children are also inconsistent. There may be an absent parent, especially the father (Scherl & Mack, 1966; Goldstein, 1972). The mother-son relationship is often conflictual and marked by an unresolved love-hate relationship (Scherl & Mack, 1966; Easson & Steinhilber, 1961; Smith, 1965; Sargent, 1962). Sometimes this conflict is exhibited by adolescents who have L-O-V-E and H-A-T-E tattoed on the fingers of each hand. Marital role conflicts also have been reported in homes with aggressive adolescents (Amanat & Able, 1973). Here one observes alliances forming where the adolescent offspring becomes the surrogate spouse for one of the parents. In extreme instances the adolescent not only replaces one of the parents, but takes his or her life as well (Smith, 1965; Hellstein & Katila, 1965; Bender, 1960).

Families in which this lethal act takes place have been studied extensively. One of the characteristics of these families is that they are often catastrophically stressed and severely disorganized. There is often severe parental sexual and/or physical abuse of the child, and the parental victim is frequently seen as a sadistic figure whom the whole family hates (Tannay, 1973).

One sees from these few dynamics that violence does not take place in a vacuum. To be sure, there are instances in which the violent act is committed under the influence of alcohol or drugs or in a psychotic state, but even here one must be aware of the dynamics involved.

DENIAL

A particular dynamic that is frequently observed in violent interactions is that of denial. Statistics on spouse and child abuse are underestimated, because more often than not such attacks go unreported and the seriousness is often denied (Steinmetz & Strauss, 1974; Kempe & Helfer, 1972). Child abusers are notorious for their use of denial. When attacks by adolescents take place in the home it is not so much that the adolescent denies, but often the parent victim is the one who employs denial. It is a common experience to hear parents minimize or deny outright that their offspring has a problem with temper, even after there has been serious physical harm. An extreme example was the case of a mother who had her back broken by her son and still, along with the father, felt that the son did not really have a problem with temper.

This kind of denial can be viewed in several ways. It may be seen as an attempt by the parent to protect, or in this instance, to overprotect the adolescent. Such silence also makes it less likely that the adolescent will have to leave home. It also protects the parents from having to admit that their own offspring physically assaulted them and, in some instances, attempted to take their life. The sense of having failed as a parent is analogous to feelings experienced by battered wives who sometimes believe they have failed as spouses. It can also be viewed as one more instance of parental neglect. Whatever purpose denial might serve in a particular family, the immediate effect is that, once again, the parents refuse to respond, neglect to set appropriate limits, and, in effect, ignore their adolescent offspring.

Some parents feel that their adolescent offspring should be given a second chance, much like the many second chances given to older perpetrators of violent crime. They are neither punished nor helped. They too are ignored in the hope that in some way all of this violent behavior will right itself. It is not only parents who employ denial; the court system and the mental health profession frequently employ this defense. Adolescents who have physically assaulted someone within or outside the home do need to be given a chance to learn how to control their behavior. This second chance demands structures and guidelines that were not present before and that the parents agree to enforce. To set limits in this manner conveys to the adolescents not only that they have committed a serious act but also that they are being taken seriously themselves. To ignore individuals, especially after they have committed a violent act, is to tell them that they are not important. The following is an example of the unwillingness of some parents to set limits.

A 17-year-old adolescent male presented with behavior problems at home and in the school. School officials and parents met on several occasions to discuss the behavior of this youngster. The parents took the attitude that their son was just "being a boy" and that there was nothing to be concerned about. Parents were asked by school authorities to begin to set limits at home. The adolescent was told that he had to be home by a certain hour. He did not comply and no action was taken by his parents. He then began to come home under the influence of alcohol. Again nothing was done. Later, on one of these evenings, when he had been drinking rather heavily, he had a serious accident with the family car. It was at this point that the adolescent himself asked his parents what he would have to do before they would take him seriously.

Such a lack of response on the part of the parents leads to feelings of helplessness within the parents and the adolescent. The parents appear incapable of changing the behavior of their son. They thus convey to him that they will not be able to assist, and, in effect, let him know that he is basically on his own. This in turn can be overpowering for the adolescent and may even lead to future acting-out behavior. It is true that adolescents need to establish a sense of independence, of self-confidence, but these goals are not easily attained when too much is asked too soon.

ABDICATION OF POWER

In homes where there is violence often one or both parents have given up their parental position. There are also many instances of overt or covert competition so that as a result both are ineffective as parents. It happens from time to time that the adolescent is forced to assume a role that rightfully belongs to one of the parents. Much stress is brought to bear on an adolescent who is emotionally dependent on parents and yet forced to assume a role and exercise a power that should be manifested by parents. One sees this happening often in overly enmeshed families where no one is allowed to really separate. In these instances the violent behavior of the adolescent offspring can be viewed as a primitive distancing measure. In one particular family the parents had been advised in the presence of the adolescent to call the police when future violence occurred. Despite this frequent admonition the parents could not bring themselves to follow this direction. On one occasion the adolescent himself fulfilled the parental responsibility and called the police on himself, telling them that he could no longer control his behavior.

FAMILY INTERACTIONAL STUDIES

Studies employing methodologies that allow for direct observational analysis aid in understanding internal family structures of delinquents. Stabenau et al. (1965) reported findings from work done with the Revealed Differences Test, the Object Sorting Test, and the Thematic Apperception Test. They were able to find definite differences among families of schizophrenics, delinquents, and normals. The delinquent families were characterized by undercontrolled affect, manipulation of family members, instability of family roles, more competitive interactions, and no clear differentiation of family leadership. Interestingly, the authors found that there was definite impairment among the parents of delinquents in their ability to conceptually abstract.

Minuchin et al. (1967) carried out extensive family interactional studies of very poor families that had more than one delinquent member. Many of the families were disorganized, black, and one-parented. The delinquents manifested a variety of antisocial behaviors, including violence. The parents tended to respond to their children's behavior in a random and inconsistent fashion. Usually, the parents attempted only to inhibit and control their children's behavior, but made no attempt to guide them. Gross deficits in family structure were noted, such as unstable father figures, one-parent families, extreme fluctuation in parental power from absolute power to helplessness, and major breakdowns in communication between parents and children.

Reiss (1967) found that families of delinquents, when compared with those of schizophrenics and normals, did not make accurate inferences of the ideas of other family members. In another study Reiss (1971) found that families of delinquents tended to be ''distance sensitive'' in that they experienced other persons in the environment as irrelevant and unrelated.

VIOLENT ADOLESCENTS

Violent adolescents themselves have been described as being defiant, physically assaultive, unsure of their roles within the family structure, and manifesting an inability to delay gratifications, plan for the future, or tolerate frustrations (Friedman, Mann, & Friedman, 1975; Offer, Marohn, & Ostrov, 1975). Another common characteristic of assaultive adolescents is poor school performance and, at times, learning disabilities (Scherl & Mack, 1966; King, 1975; Smith, 1965; Farrington & West, 1971). This often has been attributed to stress, and sociocultural and educational deprivation. Investigators focusing on delinquency in general have found evidence of organic features that could contribute to academic failure (Dehoff, 1968; Frederickson & Mulligan, 1972).

There has been more emphasis on neurological factors in adults who are violent and assaultive. One of the few studies to focus specifically on the neurological aspects of violent adolescents found a high incidence of brain damage with abnormal EEGs (Bender, 1960). Russell and Harper (1973) report 10% of their sample of assaultive adolescents as manifesting some neurological impairment.

The way we interpret our environment and our cognitive responses to that environment are highly dependent on cortical functions. It has been suggested in the literature that how we perceive ourselves and our environment may well insulate against delinquency (Reckless, Dinitz, & Kay, 1957; Reckless, Dinitz, & Murray, 1956; Scarpitti, Murray, Dinitz, & Reckless, 1962). The opposite reaction may also be seen and promotes a rationalization of delinquent behavior (Sykes & Matza, 1957). Adolescents are especially susceptible to the influence of labeling by others, and, thus, when they are labeled bad or delinquent this may enforce a self-perception of delinquency and create a self-fulfilling prophecy (Lemert, 1951; Lentz, 1966; Schwartz & Skolnick, 1964; Tannenbaum, 1938).

Shah and Roth (1974) suggest that there is much evidence that biological factors need to be considered in any adequate scientific explanation of criminal and delinquent behavior. They suggest that individuals belonging to certain population groups are greater risks for perinatal and birth complications that may result in neurological dysfunctioning. These damaged individuals further exposed to unfavorable social environments would be expected to display higher rates of deviant behaviors leading to criminal labeling.

Studies strongly suggest that learning disabilities as seen in assaultive adolescents may be associated with an organic brain dysfunction of the higher cortical areas. Other organic factors associated with delinquency in the literature have included mental retardation, minimal brain dysfunction, and certain patterns of epileptic disturbance (Jenkins & Pacella, 1943; Peterson, Quay, & Cameron, 1959). There have been a number of studies employing EEG measures in relationship with episodic aggressive behavior, but recent studies in this area have failed to distinguish aggressive from nonaggressive delinquents (Woods, 1961; Loomis, 1965; Wiener, Delano, & Klass, 1966; Loomis, Bohnert, & Huncke, 1967; Assael, Kohen-Raz, & Alpeen, 1967).

HOW VIOLENT ADOLESCENTS PRESENT

Violent adolescents, like violent adults, often appear with a generalized acknowledgment of problems with violence but are lacking in specifics. They may be aware that they are unhappy and mad much of the time, and seen by others, especially family members, as being like a "powder keg" that can go off at any moment. They may not really appreciate what precipitates their behavior. When asked what is troubling them, they respond that everything is wrong with their lives. And when asked with whom they are angry, they include everyone. It can also happen that adolescents target as the source of their pain someone or something that may not be the real source of conflict and pain for them.

An example of this was a 17-year-old adolescent male who destroyed the furniture in the home of his parents. At times of upset he had even taken Spanish decorative swords from the wall and threatened his parents. These episodes took place after he had difficulties in his relationship with his girlfriend. The parents, unaware of these difficulties, found themselves feeling helpless and confused when attempting to understand their son's behavior. For this young man it was too threatening to speak about his stormy relationship with his girlfriend. It was easier and safer for him to display anger toward his parents.

Work with violent adolescents requires much patience. The process of coming to understand what the real precipitants are is a long one. Sometimes only after long contact with the individual do we begin to see what is at the root of the behavior.

When one thinks of the amount of effort needed to master some of the more mechanical aspects of life such as walking and balance, one easily recognizes that these skills take time to learn. Some of the more profound aspects of human development also take time. One such aspect of personality development is the ability to trust. Before we can learn to trust others, we must begin to trust ourselves.

TRUST—THE BEGINNING OF CHANGE

Violent adolescents do not trust and know themselves to be untrustworthy. This is something that often is ignored in the treatment of adolescents. In an attempt to establish a relationship workers often begin by an overdisplay of trust. The adolescents know their behavior has demonstrated to any observer that they have been out of control and also realize that, because of this, they cannot trust themselves. One way to help them establish the building of trust is by the setting of limits. Realistic limits that are consistent with expectations can have a great effect. Patients who trust their therapist are able to display their emotions.

The display of anger can be viewed as a plus factor in working with violent adolescents. One can only be highly suspicious of violent individuals who never display anger in the therapy session. This can serve as a warning to the therapist that not much is going on in the therapy. Sometimes patients do not express anger in the session because they sense this is something that cannot be tolerated by the therapist. They may be forced to express this feeling in their accustomed manner outside the session and against others, such as family members.

Lack of expression of anger can also be understood as the patient's attempt to give the therapist what he or she is looking for—a nice, calm person who is developing insight. Therapists who themselves have problems in expressing anger will have difficulty in honestly allowing their patients to express such feelings. Unexpressed anger is ignored anger, and like other unexpressed emotions, takes its toll. Individuals who tell you how angry they are, even in a bellicose manner, are a lot safer to be around than those who are seething within and who continue to tell the therapist that nothing is bothering them.

In the course of working with mental health professionals the author has used videotapes of two adolescents. One of them had never committed a violent act, but in the interview graphically described how he would like to physically assault the father of his girlfriend whom he believed belittled him. His descriptions of what he would like to do included such things as breaking the father's kneecap so that he would not be able to walk and be in great pain. The other young man had actually killed two people but throughout the interview denied any hostile feelings, and went so far as to give a minisermon on the sacredness of life. This second young man presented himself as a very pleasant individual. In viewing the tapes many workers stated that they found the first adolescent to be the more dangerous. He is dangerous, to be sure, but his anger and violence are available for inspection and treatment. The second adolescent is the one who is really more dangerous because he gives no signs, no warning, and, therefore, future acts cannot easily be predicted. His history shows not only that he is capable of taking the life of another but that he actually had done so. And the best predictor of future violent behavior is a history of past violence.

CONCLUSION

The literature on juvenile delinquency must be read critically. Oftentimes there is a mix of subjects, including truants with physically assaultive adolescents, and therefore it is difficult to determine which particular group is being reported on. Rodman and Grams, in their summary of the major research in the field up to 1967, also point out that there are different types of delinquents, such as the occasional delinquent, the gang delinquent, and the maladjusted delinquent. Differences in family backgrounds have been found to vary depending upon the type of delinquency. Only a few projects reported on in the literature have systematically attempted to delineate delinquent types. Most of the literature has lumped the different kinds of delinquents together. Rodman and Grams (1967) conclude that there are many variables related to delinquency, stating that "family variables, particularly parental affection and parental discipline, are among the most important variables. It is possible, of course, that the rather clouded multi-causal picture which emerges from the research may be cleared somewhat by attention to types of delinquency rather than through dealing grossly with delinquency as a variable" (p. 209).

Even if clinicians could accurately discriminate between various groups of delinquent adolescents, we must remember that these groups cannot be considered homogeneous. Violent adolescents are first of all individuals, and any attempt at understanding must keep this in mind. Societal factors and cultural determinants have not been mentioned in this paper. These factors were not included because discussion was limited to clinical issues. However, these realities cannot be ignored if we are to understand the phenomenon of adolescent violence.

REFERENCES

Amanat, E., & Able, S. Marriage role conflicts and child psychopathology. *Adolescence*, 1973, *8* (32), 575-588.

Assael, M., Kohen-Raz, R., & Alpeen, S. Developmental analysis of EEG abnormalities in juvenile delinquents. *Diseases of the Nervous System*, 1967, *28*, 49-54.

Bender, L. Children and adolescents who have killed. *American Journal of Psychiatry*, 1960, *116*, 510-513.

Dehoff, E. Developmental and predictive characteristics of items from the Meeting Street School Screening Test. *Developmental Medicine and Child Neurology*, 1968, *10* (2), 220-232.

Doder, D. Letter from Moscow. *The Washington Post*, March 8, 1982, p. A-10.

Duncan, J.W., & Duncan, G.M. Murder in the family: A study of some homicidal adolescents. *American Journal of Psychiatry*, 1971, *127*, 1498-1502.

Easson, W.M., & Steinhilber, R.M. Murderous aggression by children and adolescents. *Archives of General Psychiatry*, 1961, *4*, 1-9.

Farrington, D., & West, D. A comparison between early delinquents and young aggressives. *British Journal of Criminology*, 1971, *11* (4), 341-358.

Frederickson, H., & Mulligan, R. *The child and his welfare.* San Francisco: Freeman, 1972.

Friedman, C.J., Mann, F., & Friedman, A.S. A profile of juvenile street gang members. *Adolescence*, 1975, *10* (40), 563-607.

Gardiner, M. *The deadly innocents.* New York: Basic Books, 1976.

Goldstein, H.S. Internal controls in aggressive children from father-present and father-absent families. *Journal of Consulting and Clinical Psychology*, 1972, *39* (3), 512.

Hamparian, D.M., Schuster, R., Dinitz, S., & Conrad, J.P. *The violent few: A study of dangerous juvenile offenders.* Lexington, Mass.: Lexington Books, 1978.

Hellstein, P., & Katila, O. Murder and other homicide by children under 15 in Finland. *Psychiatric Quarterly (Supplement)*, 1965, *39*, 54-74.

Jenkins, R., & Pacella, B. Electroencephalographic studies of delinquent boys. *American Journal of Orthopsychiatry*, 1943, *13*, 107-120.

Kalogerakis, M.G. Homicide in adolescents: Fantasy and deed. In J. Fawcett (Ed.), *Dynamics of violence.* Chicago: AMA, 1972, pp. 93-103.

Kempe, H.C., & Helfer, R.E. *Helping the battered child and his family*, Philadelphia: Lippincott, 1972.

King, C.H. The ego and the integration of violence in homicidal youth. *American Journal of Orthopsychiatry*, 1975, *45*, 134-145.

Lemert, E. *Social pathology: A systematic approach to the theory of sociopathic behavior.* New York: McGraw-Hill, 1951.

Lentz, W. Delinquency as a stable role. *Social Work*, 1966, *11* (4), 66-70.

Loomis, S. Ego abnormalities as a correlate of behavior in adolescent male delinquents. *American Journal of Psychiatry*, 1965, *121*, 1003-1006.

Loomis, S., Bohnert, P., & Huncke, S. Prediction of EEG abnormalities in adolescent delinquents. *Archives of General Psychiatry*, 1967, *17*, 494-497.

Minuchin, S., Montalvo, B., Guerney, B.G., Rosman, B.L., & Schumer, F. *Families of the slums.* New York: Basic Books, 1967.

Offer, D., Marohn, R.C. & Ostrov, E. Violence among hospitalized delinquents. *Archives of General Psychiatry*, 1975, *32*, 1180-1186.

Peterson, D., Quay, H., & Cameron, G. Personality and background factors in juvenile delinquency as inferred from questionnaire responses. *Journal of Consulting Psychology*, 1959, *23*, 395-399.

Reckless, W., Dinitz, S., & Kay, B. The selfcomponent in potential delinquency and potential nondelinquency. *American Sociological Review*, 1957, *22* (5), 566-570.

Reckless, W., Dinitz, S., & Murray, E. Self-concept as an insulator against delinquency. *American Sociological Review*, 1956, *21* (6), 744-756.

Reiss, D. Individual thinking and family interaction. Introduction to an experimental study of problem solving in families of normals, character disorders and schizophrenics. *Archives of General Psychiatry*, 1967, *16*, 80-93.

Reiss, D. Varieties of consensual experience. Contrasts between families of normals, delinquents and schizophrenics. *Journal of Nervous and Mental Disease*, 1971, *152*, 73-95.

Rodman, H., & Grams, P. Juvenile delinquency and the family: A review and discussion, Appendix L in *Task Force on Juvenile Delinquency*, the President's Commission on Law Enforcement and Administration Justice, Juvenile Delinquency and Youth Crime. Washington, D.C.: Superintendent of Documents, U.S. Government Printing Office, 1967, pp. 188-221.

Russell, O.H. & Harper, G.P. Who are our assaultive juveniles? A study of 100 cases. *Journal of Forensic Sciences*, 1973, *18*, 385-397.

Sadoff, R.L. Clinical observations on paracide. *Psychiatric Quarterly*, 1971, *45*, 65-69.

Sargent, D. Children who kill: A family conspiracy? *Social Work*, 1962, *7*, 35-42.

Scarpitti, F., Murray, E., Dinitz, S., & Reckless, W. The good boy in a high delinquency area. In M. Wolfgang L. Savitz & N. Johnson (Eds.). *The sociology of crime and delinquency*. New York: Wiley, 1962.

Scherl, D.J., & Mack, J.E. A study of adolescent matricide. *Journal of the American Academy of Child Psychiatry*, 1966, *5*, 569-593.

Schwartz, R., & Skolnick, J. Two studies of legal stigma. In H. Becker (Ed.) *The other side: Perspectives on deviance*. New York: The Free Press, 1964, pp.103-117.

Shah, S., & Roth, L. Biological and psychophysiological factors in criminality. In D. Glaser (Ed.). *Handbook of criminology*. New York: Rand McNally, 1974.

Smith, S. The adolescent murder: A psychodynamic interpretation. *Archives of General Psychiatry*, 1965, *13*, 310-319.

Stabenau, J.R., Tupin, J., Werner, M., & Pollin, W. A comparative study of families of schizophrenics, delinquents and normals. *Psychiatry*, 1965, *28*, 45-59.

Steinmetz, S.A., & Strauss, M.A. (Eds). *Violence in the family*. New York: Dodd, Mead, 1974.

Sykes, G., & Matza, D. Techniques of neutralization: A theory of delinquency. *American Sociological Review*, 1957, *22* (6), 664-670.

Tannay, E. Adolescents who kill parents—reactive paracide. *Australian and New Zealand Journal of Psychiatry*, 1973, *7*, 263-277.

Tannenbaum, F. *Crime and the community*. Boston: Ginn, 1938.

Wiener, J., Delano, J., & Klass, D. An EEG study of delinquent and nondelinquent adolescents. *Archives of General Psychiatry*, 1966, *15*, 144-150.

Woods, S. Adolescent violence and homicide: Ego disruption and the 6 and 14 dysrhythmia. *Archives of General Psychiatry*, 1961, *5*, 528-534.

7. Family Interventions from Women's Shelters

M. Ellen Traicoff, M.S.
Administrator/Clinical Supervisor
Family Violence Program
Southlake Center for Mental Health
Merriville, Indiana

Seven

THE ESTABLISHMENT OF SAFE SHELTERS FOR VICTIMS OF domestic violence is necessary if society is going to address the problem of spousal abuse. However, a refuge is not enough. Indeed, providing refuges may well contribute to maintaining the violence by exhibiting the very characteristics of the malfunctional system that produced the violence. In addition, if we identify shelter programs as being havens for the victims of domestic violence, we need to ask who the victim is. Are not all members of violent families victims?

With the advent of the increasing growth of shelter programs, we must look at what is now understood about family violence and use this knowledge to develop effective shelter programs that not only provide the necessary safety for families but also facilitate intervention in the system that produces the violence.

The purpose of this article is to describe a model shelter program that recognizes the characteristics of the violent family system and applies family systems theory in its development and ultimate delivery of services.

BACKGROUND

The shelter movement developed in the sixties. With the advent of Chiswick Women's Aid (in England) in 1971 an international trend was underway. Shelters have been established by women for women and tend to operate on the premise of women supporting women as women rather than professionals helping clients find solutions to problems (Del Martin,

1976). While each shelter has unique characteristics most shelters operate with a female, feminist-oriented staff and/or volunteers (one shelter did employ a man for the "nice male image") (Del Martin, 1976).

Most shelters are hidden, although maintaining the secret address becomes almost impossible. The general theory that seems to prevail in these "refuges" for battered women is one that is related to patriarchy theory (Dobash & Dobash, 1979). There is an identification of the battered woman as a victim not only of her spouse but also of society (Del Martin, 1976).

It is this author's contention that shelter programs that maintain secrecy perpetrate the secret game of "hide, seek, find, and beat." Programs that identify the woman as a victim of the spouse and of society may well reinforce helplessness and a sense of not being responsible. Shelters that are female operated and isolated from the community may well reinforce the notion that the problem of battered women is only a women's issue and not a community issue and therefore not a community responsibility.

In all fairness we should acknowledge that the shelter concept and the approach to dealing with the problem of battered women that existed in the sixties and into the seventies may have been necessary. It was indeed instrumental in raising the level of consciousness on the part of society with regard to the plight of battered women.

A review of the literature on family violence prior to 1980 reveals little research and perhaps is a reflection of society's lack of concern for spousal abuse. However, in recent years there has been a surge in research. A number of theories of family violence have been developed. Gelles (1980) identifies five theories of family violence:

1. resource theory
2. ecological theory
3. evolutionary theory
4. patriarchy theory

SYSTEMS THEORY AND FAMILY VIOLENCE

Straus's General Systems Theory (1973) assumes that violence between members of a family is a "systemic product" rather than a chance aberration or a product of inadequate socialization or a warped or psychotic personality. Straus views the family as a system product rather than an individual pathology.

In treatment, then, the family system, rather than the individual battered female or battering male, is seen as the basic unit. By focusing on the family system and orchestrating change within the system, change occurs in the individual members of the system (Minuchin, 1974).

There are some definite differences between functional families and dysfunctional families. Developing a shelter program for the violent family system requires identifying the characteristics of each type of family. Minuchin (1974) emphasizes that the functional family must be able to adjust when circumstances change. He further states that the continued viability of the family depends on having a sufficient range of patterns and the flexibility to utilize these when necessary.

Violent families demonstrate certain common characteristics. They are closed systems. There is a firm commitment to maintain a tight boundary between the family and the outside world. Violent families most often have strong, inflexible family rules. These can range from overt rules governing the movement of the wife to unstated rules that every family member observes. A common rule is that of secrecy. Family members may be aware of the violent behavior that takes place but not speak of "it." The battered wife herself may not confront her husband with the fact that he beat her and indeed may make excuses for him or deny the severity of the beating. In battering families there are rigid rules and roles as well as a limited capacity to cope with change as needed.

The boundaries and the roles in the battering family often are unclear and may be inappropriately reversed at various times. The expectations of family members are often unstated or inappropriately determined. Within the battering family there is often a great deal of difficulty in setting limits and following through when limits are stated. A prime example is the battering itself: the wife may never have said she would not tolerate the beating and she has passively accepted it as her lot in life. Very often when the wife does set limits, via the pressing of assault charges, she does not follow through and drops the charges. It can be argued that there are extenuating circumstances surrounding these decisions. However, generally there is a pattern of not setting limits and following through, and this can often be seen in child-rearing practices as well.

The communication system in the dysfunctional family is indirect and family members have difficulty in expressing feelings. They often make statements about what they don't want rather than what they do want. It is also assumed that one should not ask for what is wanted. There is often a blaming of others or an overblaming of self for the violent behavior that is occurring rather than an identification of mutual responsibility for the behavior.

Violent families, like all others, are complex systems. Through the use of a systems approach, predictable system changes can occur, and these in turn can result in change within individual family members (Kramer, 1980). If violent families are to be assisted we must understand the system and determine appropriate interventions in order to provide for beneficial changes throughout the system.

A MODEL SHELTER PROGRAM

With the opening of The Caring Place in 1979, Southlake Center for Mental Health (in Merriville, Indiana) became the first mental health center to operate a family violence shelter. Developed to provide immediate relief and intervention, The Caring Place provides comprehensive services for victims of family violence. (While we will use the terms "family," "wife," "husband," and "spouse" throughout this article, we consider family violence to include any violent behavior occurring between persons currently or previously involved in an intimate relationship.) Temporary shelter, crisis intervention, individual, family, and marital counseling, advocacy services, and telephone counseling are provided on a 24-hour basis by mental health professionals and trained volunteers. The Caring Place has made such services available to over one thousand women and their families.

The general philosophy of the shelter is based on a systemic theory centering on the belief that all members in a violent family are victims and in need of services. No one person is to blame. The battered wife suffers, as does the battering husband, from the stresses of daily living and family life. If children are in the household they too experience the stresses within the family caused by the violence and marital strife. To deal with the problem of family violence, all members need help in constructively effecting change in the system that produces the violent behavior. Thus, the family system is the basic unit for treatment and the focus is on understanding the relationships and effecting interventions.

The policies and procedures of The Caring Place reflect the philosophy of the program as well as the system that is being provided services. With this in mind, the shelter is an open shelter rather than a closed shelter.

The exact address of the shelter is publicized and indeed advertised. A map to the shelter is printed on the brochure. By modeling how an open system operates we are in effect "practicing what we preach."

In most cases the violent family is uninvolved in the community and often does not avail itself of the resources of that community. In the belief that family balance is a community issue, The Caring Place volunteers make an important contribution to the program and represent community support and involvement. The volunteer group provides not only volunteer service hours (36,000 hours in 3 years) but also financial support for the program.

Referrals to The Caring Place come from social service agencies such as police departments, emergency rooms, welfare departments, friends, or family. Following the initial intake process, the major focus is to provide a therapeutic climate for the woman and her children.

The atmosphere at the shelter is varied, quiet and serene at one moment and noisy and busy the next. The concept of the family unit is reinforced as women maintain responsibilities of caring for their children, rooms, laundry, etc., though they may ask for assistance if they wish. The concept of community cooperation and participation is fostered through group living involving the preparation of meals, cleanup, and general daily living tasks. Skills in interpersonal relationships are often developed as the women live together. This is important since many times the woman has been isolated from family and friends. Family contact, following the initial crisis interval, is encouraged and it is not unusual to see husbands and fathers as well as other family members visiting or having a cup of coffee with their wives and children. It is our belief that family and friends often influence a woman, both positively and negatively, in her decision regarding her marital relationship. We believe that by involving these elements of her total family system we are better able to provide the support she needs to make decisions. Very often within the safe climate of The Caring Place, all family members can view the situation in a realistic manner and make appropriate decisions.

Thus The Caring Place recognizes the need for ongoing support services as well as immediate safe housing. Emergency shelter is not enough. Counseling by specially trained mental health workers is provided to persons using the shelter or seeking help while living in the community. Individual counseling is provided for the battered spouse and the batterer. Negotiating sessions help the individuals develop ways of eliminating battering.

There is an emphasis on assisting the battered woman and/or her spouse to recognize and face current problems and then proceed with the remediation of those problems. For the woman who decides to leave the relationship there is individual counseling and social linkage.

A major concern in an open shelter is safety. During the initial assessment period it is determined what type of violence has occurred and what means of violence may be used. The assistance and cooperation of the local police department as well as area police departments are a vital component of the program.

During the time The Caring Place has been in operation there have been no injuries to clients, volunteers, or staff. Nor has there been building damage. In fact, we have maintained the same glass door since Day One. This is not to say that we have not had experience with very hostile males who see The Caring Place as a threat to their position. It is important that staff be trained in deescalating potentially violent situations and proper procedures be developed.

Conflict and struggle are necessary in family life to achieve goals and satisfaction. However, when the situation becomes destructive psychologically or physically, assistance is needed. In order to provide assistance to the family it is necessary to establish contact with all members involved, primarily the marital dyad. It is an established procedure that the batterer is contacted within 24 hours.

It has been our experience that when we make contact with the spouse we are better able to assess the system and therefore are in a better position to provide appropriate interventions. In addition, we have found that when we do not have contact with the batterer and the woman returns to the home situation, she will again be battered and will return to the shelter. The shelter does not have a limit on the number of times a woman can return. We do find that the cases in which women return more than three times are those in which we have no face-to-face contact and little phone contact with the batterer.

The contact with the spouse is made by staff and at all times the wife has the right not to have any contact with him. The initial contact is usually via telephone. Staff invite him to come in and talk. The goal is to listen to his side and convey our position that we will listen, be understanding, and work to help him. If he accepts our invitation to come in and talk, we give him the address and specific directions to The Caring Place. He is also given the telephone number in case he can't find us. If he refuses, he is invited to call back or it is suggested that he will be called at a later time. If the spouse is initially hostile we are very patient and understanding of his need to ventilate. If he threatens to come in violently, we inform him that we will not tolerate violent behavior. However, if he wants to come in we will give him specific directions. Usually, this is a new response and often results in silence while he wonders what to do next.

The spouse is seen at the shelter. There are, of course, times when the spouse will attempt to control the situation. Since this has worked in the past, he will expect it to work now. It is important to be firm, set limits, and clearly identify the behavior expected and not expected. The consequences of his negativeness are clearly communicated. When necessary, police action is taken, arrests are made, and charges are filed. Follow-through is important. Very often no one has responded to the behavior in this manner and as a result police action is seldom needed. The violent spouse has often been seen by others as being all-powerful and is generally described as being a person no one can control. Usually, the wife has felt helpless in dealing with even threats of violent behavior. By seeing that the violent behavior is controllable she is reinforced in the feeling that she is not helpless. With the control of the violent behavior both the battered wife and her spouse can begin to look at the violence in their relationship and determine how to eliminate the violent behavior.

The majority of families seen at the shelter are not receptive to the idea of counseling services. We have found that when follow-up counseling services are provided at the shelter the individuals and family are more receptive. When we look at the family's process* in terms of establishing relationships outside the family system, we can better understand the difficulty in referring individual and family for follow-up counseling with outside agencies. Although it is important to establish therapeutic services that provide immediate control of the violent behavior, it is equally important to provide the supportive ongoing services that will assist in effective and lasting change in the system.

CASE ILLUSTRATIONS

The following cases illustrate the value of recognizing the system being served and how effective interventions can bring about change in the system and individuals.

---

* A family's process is defined as the manner in which the family systematically communicates and interacts within the family system as well as outside the system.

Case A

A case that illustrates the need for contact with all elements of the system and the need to penetrate the boundaries that surround and help maintain the violent behavior is that of Belinda, who returned to the shelter five times. Each time unsuccessful efforts were made to contact her spouse. Belinda's first stay was 2 days. She decided, against staff advice, to return home. Her second stay was 4 days. Again efforts to reach the spouse were unsuccessful. She returned. This time staff was able to arrange to have phone contact with her. We later found that these phone calls were monitored by her spouse. However, she identified these calls as being a "life line." Belinda returned for the third time and stayed 7 days. During this time she decided to file charges. However, Belinda decided to return home again and dropped the charges. Staff worked with her on how she could maintain herself in the system she was choosing not to leave. Contact with Belinda was maintained and during her fifth stay she was able to objectively determine her goals and implement them. Contact with her spouse was never accomplished.

Case B

In the case of Cindy one initially might question involving the batterer. Cindy came in following a severe beating by her boyfriend. She was very firm about leaving and had filed charges. She stayed 2 days and she and her children returned home. Staff had attempted to contact the boyfriend, Len, without success. The couple was not married and the house was in Cindy's name. Shortly after she returned home Len began to harass her, breaking windows and even slashing her tires. Police were called; however, he was always gone. Cindy returned to The Caring Place. This time staff was able to contact the boyfriend and he came in. Cindy was able to give him a clear direct message, which was backed up by the presence of staff. The message was that any harassment would be documented and charges would be filed and Cindy was not alone.

Case C

In the case of Bill and Mary, contact with the batterer resulted in Bill coming to The Caring Place and dealing with his violent behavior. Both Bill and Mary wanted to continue the relationship and wanted to stop the beatings. During Mary's 2-week stay she and Bill participated in individual as well as couple counseling. Each became aware of how they contributed to the dysfunctioning of their relationship. The couple negotiated the condition under which Mary would return home. Both agreed to short-term marital therapy following Mary's return home. During this time they worked out a number of issues and no violence was reported. Both agreed to discontinue marital therapy. Three months later Mary returned to the shelter. Although Bill had not beaten her she had felt significantly threatened and needed to seek a safe climate. Bill was contacted and the process was repeated. The couple agreed to marital therapy. They stayed in therapy 8 weeks. Four months later we received a call from Bill. He stated that things were "getting tight" and he thought he and Mary should come in for counseling.

This is a couple who had never received counseling services and initially were resistive. Bill had said, "What's the good of just talking?" Because of our policy of contacting spouses and the availability of more than just shelter services this couple was able to learn new ways of relating. Follow-up indicates that the violent behavior is not recurring. More important, this couple knows that if they need assistance they can come in for help before violence is the only method available for resolution.

REFERENCES

Del Martin, M. *Battered wives.* San Francisco: Glide Publications, 1976.

Dobash, R., & Dobash, R. *Violence against wives.* New York: Free Press, 1979.

Gelles, R. Violence in the family: A review of research in the seventies. *Journal of Marriage and the Family,* November 1980, pp. 873–884.

Kramer, C. *Becoming a family therapist.* New York: Human Sciences Press, 1980.

Minuchin, S. *Families and family therapy.* Cambridge, Mass.: Harvard University Press, 1974.

Straus, M. *Violence in the family.* New York: Dodd, Mead, 1973.

8. Using Cognitive and Systems Intervention in the Treatment of Marital Violence

Richard C. Bedrosian, Ph.D.
Massachusetts Center for Cognitive Therapy
Westborough, Massachusetts

Eight

THE GOAL OF THIS PAPER IS TO ILLUSTRATE HOW TECHNIQUES derived from cognitive therapy can be blended with systems interventions in order to treat domestic violence. The author assumes that only by combining interventions aimed at both the intra- and inter-personal levels can a therapist produce long-term changes in a violent marriage. For the sake of convenience, the following presentation is subdivided into sections on systems and cognitive interventions. Nonetheless, the two types of treatment strategies are continuously intertwined in the author's clinical work.

SYSTEMS ISSUES AND INTERVENTIONS

The following draws heavily upon the influence of Haley (1963, 1976), Aponte & Van Deusen (1981), Minuchin (1974), and the Palo Alto Group (Watzlawick, Beavin, & Jackson, 1967).

Engagement in Treatment

The therapist should exert considerable energy in assessing and modifying the marital system which spawns and supports the violent behavior. Clearly, members of violent marriages arrive in the consulting room in differing states of readiness for treatment. Seldom do both spouses show the same or similar levels of motivation for treatment, commitment to the marriage, willingness to introspect, and so forth. Different types of motivational configurations may appear at the initial interview.

1. The husband comes to therapy in response to an ultimatum from his wife, but for a variety of reasons is unenthusiastic at best about treatment. Some men may deceive themselves regarding the nature of the violence problem (''It was just the booze talking'') or assume that they can simply *decide* never to be violent again, without acquiring additional coping skills or a deeper understanding of the problem. For some men, therapy (along with police calls, restraining orders, involvement of in-laws, etc.) is but one of a series of humiliations to be endured as a result of a violent episode. Without changes in the marriage, such humiliations only serve as additional provocations for subsequent cycles of conflict between the spouses. The husband may believe that he is about to be blamed for *all* the family problems by the mental health professional who is *colluding* with his wife.

2. The husband comes to therapy as part of a general attitude of abasement toward the wife, who accompanies him to treatment but indicates that what he has offered her is ''too little too late.'' At first blush, the therapist will find it difficult to determine whether the wife is truly on her way out of the marriage or is waiting to see if the husband will change in some manner. The wife who stays with an abusing husband after complaining of his behavior to police, family, friends, and/or social service agencies may find herself in a position of intense triangulation. On the one hand, she may wish to preserve whatever strengths exist in the marriage, or she may be terrified of being alone. On the other hand, she does not wish to alienate friends or family members who have offered her support during the violent episode(s), but negative reactions from others are inevitable if she remains in the marriage.

The husband, meanwhile, may pursue treatment only as long as he sees a chance of preserving the marriage by doing so. The husband whose motivation for treatment stems primarily from a wish to placate his wife will also find it hard to sustain interest in therapy when and if her attitude toward him softens. Similarly, the husband whose posture is strictly a conciliatory one will find it hard to drop his ''nice guy'' persona long enough to address crucial issues in the marriage, particularly those which involve anger toward his wife.

3. The couple comes to therapy primarily due to the prompting of an agency or a significant other who has become involved in the domestic violence. Husband and wife bicker angrily during the initial office visit, while neither one appears motivated either to change or to leave the relationship. At the outset, one or both spouses may threaten the other

with terminating therapy. The partners in such a marriage are certainly poor candidates for treatment, although the therapist might see such a couple in an attempt to *induce readiness for treatment*. In making this type of decision the therapist must balance the potential benefits to the couple, to the children (if there are any in home), and to the community, against the very real psychic costs incurred by spending time with angry, abusive, unmotivated individuals.

In order to set the stage for treatment, the therapist will need to communicate the following ideas in words and gestures that will be in keeping with the couple's communicational style:

1. Since it presents a potential danger to life and limb, controlling the husband's violent behavior is the first priority of treatment. A strong stance by the wife, including her commitment to leaving the home and/or using legal channels if necessary, is *vital* to the husband's development of greater self-control. The therapist joins with the wife but *relabels* her behavior as an indication of loyalty to and concern for her husband.

2. If the husband develops better self-control, he will then be able to more effectively raise some of the issues he finds in the marriage, since he will have stepped out from ''behind the eight ball.'' On the other hand, every time he behaves in a violent manner, he frees his wife from the obligation of examining her contribution to the distressed marriage. Although the therapist joins with the husband in this maneuver, his repeated references to violence maximize the wife's tendency to cooperate.

3. Each spouse is responsible for his or her own behavior, regardless of the provocations involved. The therapist assumes that each spouse has contributed more or less equally to the marital problems and will work to short-circuit all attempts at blaming during the session. He or she regrets that it will be necessary at times to antagonize one or both spouses through insistence on the acceptance of personal responsibility. The therapist thereby attempts to inoculate the couple against subsequent resistance to treatment.

4. Husband and wife need to realize that *together*, they have created a highly dysfunctional marriage, and that treatment will work only if each of them is highly motivated to change. This maneuver aims to join the couple together, while eliciting postures and statements favorable to therapy.

Models

Since so many spouses in violent marriages were reared in abusive homes, it is useful to discuss the family of origin of each spouse. A typical example involved an abusing husband of French Canadian ancestry, whose father and older brother had regularly beaten him as a youth. As a teen-ager, he had been arrested at his father's request following a dispute in the home. His brother bailed him out of jail and promptly beat him. Thereafter, the young man took refuge with his fiancée's family. The wife, meanwhile, modeled herself after her long-suffering mother, who tolerated her chronic alcoholic husband in silence up until the time he drank himself into an early grave.

Although insight per se does not generate new behaviors or coping strategies, the review of pertinent historical material provides spouses with an understanding of how they are "primed" to utilize violence or tolerate abuse in a marital relationship. Further, the discussion of familial influences allows the spouses to empathize with one another to a greater extent, as they view the abuse problem in a context that deemphasizes blaming.

Alcohol Abuse

Clinical experience indicates that it is crucial for the therapist to assess carefully the role alcohol abuse plays in the complaint of domestic violence. Alcohol intake tends to disinhibit dominant violent responses while it prevents the individual from utilizing more creative solutions to conflict. The therapist must decide whether one or both spouses require treatment for alcohol abuse (up to and including inpatient detoxification) prior to or concurrent with any other therapeutic efforts. It is reasonable to assume that even the most well-motivated couple will continue to be at substantial risk as long as an ongoing pattern of alcohol abuse exists, particularly on the part of the abusing spouse.

The significant role of alcohol is seen in the following case: An abusing husband and his wife began treatment following a violent incident during which both spouses had been intoxicated. Both spouses minimized the extent of their alcohol problems and, typically, withheld information from the therapist. After six or seven sessions, the couple withdrew from therapy against the therapist's advice, and maintained a bitter standoff for several months thereafter. The husband increased his alcohol consumption as he became more and more depressed. Following an auto accident with suicidal overtones and another violent episode with his wife, the man finally accepted a referral to an inpatient alcoholism program. His wife, meanwhile, claimed she was moving to terminate the marriage, but continued drinking and postponing any decisions.

Some couples may not show an ongoing pattern of alcohol abuse, but may use drinking as a means of dramatizing concerns they cannot address at other times. This process occurs most frequently when one of the spouses lacks assertive skills. Some spouses report that they *consciously decide* to drink in order to get the courage to vent some long-suppressed dissatisfactions; many spouses can learn to recognize such a pattern with practice. The therapist's task in such instances is to facilitate the development of more appropriate assertive skills, while inoculating the individual against the dysfunctional cognitions ("Don't rock the boat," "It's not important enough to bother with," etc.) that inhibit assertive behavior. The therapist needs to acknowledge in advance that increased assertiveness on the part of one spouse will produce short-term increases in stress for the other spouse. However, the therapist can also emphasize that in the long run improvement in assertive skills will benefit *both* partners, in that it will serve to prevent violent episodes and the chronic unresolved conflicts which breed them.

Alcohol intake is virtually imbedded in the social contexts of many couples. A couple may find as they analyze their life style that drinking has become an integral part of nearly all of their social and recreational activities. As the spouses progress in treatment to the point where their relationship provides more satisfaction or mutual trust, they can begin to evaluate *together* their friendships and their leisure pursuits. Partners can work together to avoid certain individuals or contexts, such as other couples who drink heavily and play kissing games at parties, that have generated difficulty in the past. Likewise, couples may need the therapist's assistance in learning how to have fun together without the use of alcohol.

Defusing Conflict

When couples arrive in treatment in a state of crisis, the therapist may need to be quite directive in suggesting steps that can be taken to attenuate conflict. It may be necessary, for example, for the couple to initiate or maintain a temporary separation during the first few weeks of treatment.

Periods of contact would then occur under predictable conditions (e.g., in the therapist's office) in order to maximize the chances for developing improved interaction patterns.

As long as the level of overt conflict is high, the therapist should structure the treatment hour carefully. A few glimpses into the couple's natural communication style are satisfactory for diagnostic purposes. It is not helpful, however, to allow the highly dysfunctional couple to perseverate in their destructive communications at length in the session. As soon as possible, therefore, the therapist should begin to block destructive processes such as blaming, coercion, obsessive review of prior misdeeds, "mind reading," and so on. A typical exchange in treatment would proceed as follows:

W: I can't stand the way you (husband) are always pushing me to lose weight. You're making me depressed.

H: But, Judy, the doctor said your phlebitis could cripple you unless you took some weight off. You're causing me to worry—how can I work with this on my mind?

Th: You're both blaming one another for what's going on in your own thoughts . . .

H: (Interrupts) But wouldn't you feel the same way if your wife was sick and overweight?

Th: Yes, I would be concerned. Tell me, has she ever lost weight because you insisted on it?

H: No.

Th: What happens when you insist on it?

H: She seems determined to stay heavy.

Th: So you're telling me it doesn't work when you try to *force* her to do things.

H: Right.

Th: (To wife) And how does your husband respond when you insist that he gets more overtime work?

W: He says, "Yeah, yeah," then he ignores me, and then he blows up, which he has no right to do, because I'm just trying to help him.

Th: So when you each try to force one another to do things, the only result you see is that both of you just get more and more aggravated. That's why I'm going to stop you in here whenever I see you taking responsibility for the other person, *because it doesn't work*. Also, I know the two of you do treat each other pretty badly at times, but in the long run only *you* can make yourself less depressed and only *you* can make yourself less anxious.

The preceding exchange may need to be repeated dozens of times before highly dysfunctional partners will begin to change their style of interaction even slightly. Even the most rigid spouses can acknowledge eventually that their tactics are not working, regardless of the accuracy of the content involved. In the early stages of treatment, the therapist will play a more central role in the session, as he or she disengages the couple and blocks escalating interactions. As the therapist teaches the spouses to monitor and correct their own communications, the therapist can begin to play a less central role.

Boundaries

It seems virtually impossible to treat an abusing marriage successfully without modifying the larger family context, even if such a modification occurs in an indirect way. Likewise, it is impossible to discuss the symptom of domestic violence without considering the dysfunctional family structures that may accompany it.

The therapist may diagnose diffuse spouse subsystem boundaries, associated with weak marital bonding and minimal intimacy between partners, from the following types of observations:

1. Lack of sustained one-to-one contact between spouses without the presence of children, friends, or extended family.
2. Lack of common friends and activities.
3. Lack of consensus regarding the handling of children and extended family relationships.
4. Stable crossgenerational coalitions that exclude one spouse (e.g., husband allies with his mother against wife, wife sides with son against the husband, and so on).
5. Overprotectiveness of or overaccessibility to children.
6. Persistent "leakage" of sensitive details of the marital relationship to significant others.
7. Affairs, public quarrels, or other attempts at triangulation.

None of the phenomena just described necessarily *cause* domestic violence; indeed some will undoubtedly occur *as a result* of spouse abuse.

The presence of diffuse spouse subsystem boundaries suggests that interventions of the following types may be useful:

1. Scheduling one-to-one time between the spouses at first for the purpose of building intimacy (it may be dysfunctional for the couple to

expect to have *fun* together at the outset), later for the purpose of sharing mastery and/or pleasure activities together.

2. Building (or rebuilding) a shared peer support network.

3. Developing greater teamwork in solving childrearing and extended family difficulties.

4. Inoculating spouses against irrational anxiety regarding their children.

5. Maintaining regular periods of disengagement from children.

6. Identifying the *costs* of triangulation and assisting the couple in resisting the temptation to induct others into the marital conflicts.

From a cognitive perspective, it is impossible to implement such behavioral interventions without evoking and discussing the spouse's interpretations, expectations, and beliefs about intimacy along the way. Cognitions and behaviors are linked together in a continuous feedback loop such that new behaviors disconfirm dysfunctional cognitions, while changed thinking stimulates more adaptive actions.

COGNITIVE THERAPY

The cognitive model of psychopathology assumes that the patient's idiosyncratic interpretations, expectations, and basic assumptions trigger unpleasant affective states, undesirable behaviors, and other symptoms of psychological distress (Beck, 1976). Cognitive therapy procedures have been developed for a wide range of clinical problems, such as depression (Beck, Rush, Shaw, & Emery, 1979), agoraphobia (Coleman, 1981), and anger (Novaco, 1978). To date, a number of research studies support claims for the efficacy of cognitive therapy with various clinical problems (e.g., Hollon, Beck, Bedrosian, & Young, 1979; Novaco, 1976; Rush, Beck, Kovacs, & Hollon, 1977). Interested readers may wish to consult various source materials that detail basic cognitive therapy principles (Beck, Rush, Shaw, & Emery, 1979; Bedrosian & Beck, 1980), applications of cognitive therapy to diverse clinical problems and populations (Emery, Hollon, & Bedrosian, 1981; Kendall & Hollon, 1979), and specific cognitive approaches to anger control (Novaco, 1978). Recently, cognitive therapists have described how their techniques can be integrated with procedures aimed at modifying marital and/or family systems (Beck, 1980; Bedrosian, 1981).

It is assumed that a strong *collaborative* relationship between therapist and patient is a necessary component of effective cognitive therapy. Contrary to misconceptions of cognitive therapy (Ledwidge, 1978), the cognitive therapist does not simply get the patient to "change his or her mind" through the use of didactic techniques. The therapist and patient(s) work *together* to identify the connections between specific thoughts, unpleasant emotions, and undesirable behaviors. Likewise, once the salient cognitions have been identified, the therapist and patient collaborate to evaluate the validity and/or utility of each belief or interpretation.

Cognitions and Spouse Abuse

When they enter treatment, most abusing spouses are aware of the provocations and the resulting emotions that lead to violent behavior, but few patients recognize the cognitions which mediate the relationships between external events and subsequent affect and behavior. Moreover, few spouses are aware of the powerful influence exerted by their interpretations and attitudes upon their marital relationships.

The cognitive therapy literature cited earlier contains descriptions of various methods for assessing dysfunctional cognitions. Reporting on one's thought processes is a skill that a patient can learn during the therapy hour. The therapist may ask the patient to reexperience the troublesome situations, and to reveal the automatic thoughts associated with the incident. Similarly, problem situations that involve interpersonal interactions can be recreated in the interview through the use of role playing. The "ideal" cognitive therapy patient will begin recording his or her dysfunctional cognitions *in vivo* between sessions. The majority of patients who record their dysfunctional thoughts use the "Triple Column" technique (Beck et al., 1979), which requires that the patient:

1. Briefly describe an upsetting incident.
2. Identify the emotions associated with it.
3. List the corresponding automatic thoughts.
4. Provide rational responses to the dysfunctional ideation.

Since not all patients, particularly those who lack psychological sophistication, will comply with homework assignments, the therapist may need to confine his or her assessment strategies and treatment interventions to those that can be implemented during the treatment session.

As part of a complete assessment, the therapist aims to learn as much as possible about the setting in which anger-inducing cognitions occur, as well as the frequency and duration of the dysfunctional thoughts. Novaco (1978) outlines a comprehensive method for assessing anger problems. In addition to obtaining information regarding the parameters of violent behavior, the therapist also needs to determine whether the patient already possesses any successful mechanisms for coping with anger. It may be possible for the therapist to build upon coping skills that are already in the patient's repertoire.

The following is an illustrative case. A husband became enraged and violent after his wife had stayed out much later than she had originally planned. Previous abusive episodes had also occurred on evenings when the wife had stayed out late. Interestingly, the husband had no problem tolerating the wife's absence on other occasions, since she regularly vacationed with her mother and sister. A month prior to the current abusive episode, the wife had narrowly escaped serious injury in a spectacular auto accident caused by another driver. The therapist attempted to elicit the automatic thoughts that had preceded the husband's violence.

Th: What were you thinking when your wife came home?

H: I don't remember. It was just bullshit.

Th: Okay. Can you remember where you were and what you were thinking when you first realized she was late?

H: Well, I was sitting downstairs on the couch. The first thing I thought was, what if she had an accident?

Th: How did you feel then?

H: Scared. I remembered her accident.

Th: So then what did you think when she came home?

H: First I was relieved. Then I thought, she's always doing this to me, she doesn't give a shit about me, all I do is work my tail off for this family, and this is the thanks I get.

Th: And then you hit the ceiling.

Through a variety of similar experiences in therapy, the husband was able to recognize that his episodes of violence and extreme anger generally sprang from the same sources. He would experience fear as he speculated on the possible threats to his wife's safety, and disappointment as he recognized her failure to call him. Fear and disappointment would quickly turn to anger, however, as he reinterpreted his wife's actions as *personally directed* at him and went on to ruminate about her history of previous transgressions. Such rumination only served to escalate his anger (and the accompanying autonomic responses) to the point where he was no longer able to control himself.

The husband was slow to engage in treatment, to say the least. During the initial office visit, he stormed out to his car after his wife opened the session with a series of disparaging remarks about him. The therapist followed him out and was able to coax him back inside by saying, ''I think your point of view is probably important, but if you leave now, I'll only get one side of the story.'' On another occasion, the man walked into the consulting room, looked at his watch, and announced to therapist, ''This is my last session. I'm sick of this bullshit. You've got two minutes to say what you want to say, then I'm leaving.'' He promptly walked out of the office, forcing his wife to take a taxi home. Both incidents recounted above began with experiences of rejection by the wife, which the husband quickly converted into anger. Only the therapist's willingness to ''walk the second mile,'' by maintaining contact with the man during these irrational outbursts succeeded in engaging him in treatment.

The major themes that emerged in the husband's dysfunctional cognition were:

1. The tendency to *personalize*, to interpret the actions of others as being aimed at him.
2. *Rigid, all-or-nothing expectations* of himself and others (e.g.,''If I make a mistake, I'm worthless,'' or ''If my wife lets me down once, it means she doesn't love me'').
3. The tendency to *overgeneralize* and *catastrophize* as a result of negative experiences (e.g., ''My marriage and my entire life are worthless because my wife and I fought again last night'').
4. Persistent *mislabeling* of affective states (e.g., ''If I feel sad or disappointed, someone must be to blame, and should be punished'').
5. Repeated *negative predictions*, which prevented him from following through on behavioral changes (e.g., ''There's no point in going fishing, since I know I won't enjoy myself anyway'').
6. Inability to prevent *rumination*, once anger-inducing cognitions began.

The reader will note that the ideational themes just described trap the individual in a vicious cycle. To paraphrase songwriter Paul Simon, the typical patient hears what he or she wants to hear and disregards the rest. Data that disconfirm dysfunctional ideas are consistently ignored or discounted. In the meantime, persistently high levels of emotional arousal further inhibit the development of new ideational patterns or behavioral responses. Continual rumination only exacerbates the negative affect.

Like many abusing spouses, the patient discussed above struggled nearly as much with depression as he did with anger. Clearly, his cognitions reflected the negative view of the self, the world, and the future so typically observed in the depressed patient. Some men evidently learn quite early to ward off depressogenic cognitions and depressive affect by externalizing blame and picking a fight. Once an abusing husband learns to curb his anger, treatment may then focus on self-esteem, perfectionism, hopelessness, anhedonia, and other issues associated with the underlying depression. This patient once observed, ''I never realized before that I had so many other feelings besides anger, or that I was so down on myself.''

As treatment proceeds, the therapist will also assess the dysfunctional cognitions of the abused spouse, which will often interlock in a pathogenic manner with the ideation of the abusing partner. The wife of the patient discussed in the preceding paragraphs revealed the following ideational themes:

1. A pervasive sense of *helplessness* (e.g., ''Nothing I say or do affects my husband in any way'') which inhibited the recognition of her negative impact on others and justified the use of passive-aggressive interpersonal strategies.
2. *Chronically low self-esteem* (e.g., ''I don't deserve to be happy''), which prevented her from sustaining appropriate assertive behavior.
3. Persistent *misattribution of responsibility* (e.g., ''If someone is angry at me, it must be my fault,'' or ''It's my job to bring my husband and my son closer together'').
4. *All-or-nothing expectations of relationships* (e.g., ''If I fulfill one request of my husband, then he'll begin to dominate me again'').
5. *Dysfunctional rules for the prevention of psychological pain* (e.g., ''If I withdraw, my husband won't be able to hurt me'').

The wife's cognitions served to maintain her status as a helpless victim while ensuring that attempts at more assertive behavior were accompanied by high levels of guilt. Meanwhile, her fear of further suffering at her husband's hands kept her at such a distance from him that communication about the critical issues in the relationship was virtually nonexistent.

Cognitive Interventions

Cognitive therapy utilizes treatment techniques that stem from a variety of sources. What defines a given treatment strategy as "cognitive" is not the use of a particular technique, but the *intent* of the practitioner, namely *to modify the ideation that accompanies symptoms of psychological distress*. The therapist will need to tailor the treatment strategies to the needs of the particular individual or couple. Readers who wish more extensive exposure to cognitive interventions should consult the relevant literature previously cited, particularly the selections by Novaco (1978).

Cognitive interventions and relationship interventions should not be seen as mutually exclusive. Relationship issues often surface during the investigation of dysfunctional cognitions, and vice versa. Likewise, the cognitions of both spouses should function as grist for the therapeutic mill.

Distancing and Hypothesis Testing

Through the process of self-observation, the individual begins to realize that his or her interpretations are not necessarily accurate. The therapist's consistent message is: Look for the evidence before you accept your ideas as *facts*. Partners in intimate relationships consistently engage in "mind reading"; they anticipate one another's moods, motivations, and evaluations. During conjoint sessions, the therapist has the opportunity to encourage the spouses to check the validity of their assumptions about one another directly, as the following dialogue illustrates.

W: He leaves all the discipline of Ricky up to me, because he probably doesn't want any more to do with him.

Th: You're telling me what your husband wants. Why don't you check that out with him before we go any further.

W: (To husband) Well, isn't that how you feel?

H: Not exactly. I was down on myself for the way I've been handling him, and I figured you were too. I just don't want to lose my cool with him like I used to.

W: But I thought you'd been doing better with him.

Th: So without checking, you both *assumed* you knew what the other person was thinking.

Every instance of disconfirmation aids in disengaging the individual from his or her dysfunctional cognitions. The therapist enables the patient(s) to set up "experiments" to evaluate various beliefs but takes care to anticipate both positive and negative outcomes. The patient can then view the behavior experiment as a learning experience, regardless of the outcome. The following example illustrates how the therapist sets up a task as a "no lose" situation, after eliciting the partner's cognitions.

H: We have absolutely nothing in common.

Th: What makes you say that?

H: I love the outdoors, but my wife would rather be dead than be caught on a snowmobile or a pair of skis.

Th: (To wife) Is that so?

W: Yes, I love antiques, but I've only been able to get my husband to a flea market once in the past few years, and then he begged me to go home early. Now I just go alone or with my sister.

Th: What did you do together when you were dating and during the early years of your marriage?

H: We loved going out to eat, Italian food, Chinese food, anything different. But we just stopped.

Th: What do you think would happen if you went out together for a dinner date?

W: We probably wouldn't have anything to say to each other.

H: Yeah, it could be a long night.

Th: Yes, it could be. But when we started this discussion, you both assured me that you had *nothing* in common. Now it looks like at one time you did share some interests. I'd like you to try a dinner date this week *as an experiment.* Let's see what happens. If you enjoy it, fine. If not, then we'll have a better opportunity to find out what holds you back from enjoying yourselves.

It should be noted that patients with long-term difficulties seldom restructure their beliefs as a result of one or two disconfirmatory experiences. The therapist can expect to address the same issues repeatedly, in many different ways, until the patient recognizes that he or she consistently distorts information in a certain manner, in certain situations. Once this recognition occurs, the patient can begin to dispute and/or interrupt the disturbing ideas.

A most effective distancing technique involves the judicious use of humor by the therapist. Partners who can learn to laugh at themselves acquire a powerful tool for defusing subsequent anger reactions. Moreover, the mirth response creates a positive affective tone upon which the therapist can build subsequent interventions. The author is fond of citing episodes of television shows, or instances of his own or other's dysfunctional behaviors that parallel the experiences of his patients. Characters such as Archie Bunker or Ralph Kramden of the ''Honeymooners'' are particularly fruitful sources of material, since they often reflect the self-centered, ultimately childish behavior of the abusing spouse. Since humor in the session can backfire in so many ways, therapists should utilize it only when they have a good grasp of the communicational and cognitive styles of the spouses involved.

Decatastrophizing

Abusing spouses consistently overmagnify the significance of upsetting situations. The therapist can assist the patient to reevaluate the relative importance of anger-producing episodes in a number of ways. The therapist may ask the spouse to move forward in time 10 or 20 years, then estimate the impact of the provocation, or to rate the importance of the situation relative to other significant life events. Another option involves providing patients with an opportunity to review their cognitions some time after the anger associated with a particular event has subsided, as the following example illustrates.

> A couple arrived late for a treatment session looking haggard and distressed. The husband was enraged because his wife's late departure from work prevented him from stopping off at a hardware store on the way to therapist's office, as he had originally planned. As he described it, the missed store visit set him hopelessly behind in his household tasks. Moreover, he stated that his wife's tardiness reflected her total lack of motivation to improve their relationship, and signaled the impending demise of their marriage. Although the husband's high level of arousal and agitation seemed to preclude the possibility of an immediate intervention, the therapist dutifully wrote down his comments for later use. During the next treatment session, the therapist reviewed the written record with the husband, who by then was open to reevaluating his dysfunctional conclusions.

Anger as a Cue

As Novaco (1978) points out, individuals can learn to utilize anger and/or anger-inducing cognitions as cues to engage in alternative coping strategies. Such strategies can include rational responses (see subsequent section), thought-stopping or distraction techniques (see subsequent section), or adaptive assertive responses. Alternative responses can be developed and rehearsed in the treatment session through the use of role playing (with or without the spouse taking part) or imagery.

During any kind of insession rehearsal procedure, the therapist continuously monitors the patient's cognitions as he or she works to master the new behaviors. Working through the dysfunctional cognitions that prevent the development of new skills is as crucial as the acquisition of the skills themselves. For example, a patient may perform very well at an assertiveness role play, but may think, "I'll never be able to do this outside," or "It's wrong to make such a big deal about minor issues." Clearly, the patient will never behave differently in interpersonal situations as long as he or she holds such self-defeating beliefs.

A major goal with abusing husbands is to teach them to express the themes of sadness, disappointment, rejection, and helplessness, which so often precede the experience of anger. Most husbands can learn that the consequences for expressing the so-called tender emotions to their wives in a nonaccusatory manner are far more positive than anticipated. For example, a husband persistently antagonized his wife by behaving in a jealous manner (e.g., insinuating that he was afraid to leave her alone with his friends or interrogating her about the attractiveness of the men with whom she worked). When more relaxed, the husband acknowledged that he had no reason to doubt his wife's loyalty. The accusations and innuendoes occurred at times when he felt incompetent, unlovable, or unattractive, often as a result of experiences that had nothing to do with the marriage. When he began to say, "I'm hurting," "I'm lonely," or "I need to talk about what happened at work today," he found his wife to be supportive, attentive, and affirming.

Rational Responses

With practice, patients can learn to challenge their own dysfunctional cognitions. Table 8-1 contains a sampling of rational responses and the associated dysfunctional cognitions. It should be stressed that the therapist does not "spoon feed" the rational responses to the patient. Rational responses develop as a result of the learning experiences provided in the course of therapy. Since an effective rational response requires at least a modest degree of belief from the patient, one or two responses may reflect an entire session of therapeutic work.

Table 8-1 Examples of Dysfunctional Cognitions (DC)
and Corresponding Rational Responses (RR)

DC: My wife is late again. I won't stand for this. This is one more sign that she doesn't love me.	*RR:* Her lateness isn't necessarily directed at me personally. Anyway, it's not the end of the world. She shows me in other ways she loves me.
DC: Why bother trying? I don't deserve to be happy after the way I've treated my family.	*RR:* The bad things I've done don't make me a bad person. Besides, it's not too late for me to treat them better. Rehashing the past only makes me feel bad.
DC: My wife would probably choose those educated guys from the office over me. That bitch!	*RR:* This is the way I think when something else is bothering me. Don't blame her!
DC: I screwed up at work again. Everybody knows I'm a big failure.	*RR:* One mistake doesn't make me a failure. No one's perfect.

Note. Multiple rational response options are offered for each group of dysfunctional cognitions.

The ability to generate rational responses during an actual stressful situation and thereby decrease emotional arousal represents the end point of a learning process that begins with the patient's identification of his or her maladaptive thoughts. By emphasizing that the acquisition of rational responses is a slow, incremental process, the therapist avoids giving the patient unrealistic expectations, and prevents the procedure from taking on a magical or mechanistic flavor. Further, the patient is forewarned that initially the rational responses may be difficult to produce and to believe.

In the beginning, the therapist and the patient jointly formulate and rehearse the rational responses in the treatment session. After practicing in the session, the patient's first task is to produce rational responses to thoughts that have already been recorded on the daily log. If he or she can think of the responses during an actual stressful situation, so much the better, but this would be unrealistic as an initial goal. The therapist may wish to present the following analogy to the patient: A child may be able to dribble a basketball behind his or her back when practicing in the schoolyard, but will freeze up at first in a real game. As the new skill becomes more automatic through repetition it can be performed effectively during the stress of an actual game. As Table 8-1 illustrates, rational responses can address the *utility* of pursuing a particular line of thought, as well as the *validity* of the particular cognitions.

Thought-Stopping and Distraction

At times, the abusing spouse may find it useful to simply stop the anger-inducing thoughts or to engage his attention as fully as possible on other matters. The cognitive therapy sources cited earlier contain a variety of thought-stopping and distraction techniques. It is a good idea to give patients the choice of whether to work on instituting such procedures, since some individuals find the techniques refreshingly concrete and straightforward and others perceive them as simplistic, gimmicky, and ultimately demeaning.

Reducing Arousal Level

The abusing spouse often experiences a high level of arousal which lowers the threshold for anger responses. Both behavioral and cognitive interventions can serve to reduce tension and irritability. Deep muscle relaxation, imagery techniques, and aerobic exercise (e.g., swimming, running, racquetball, and the like) all reduce the individual's resting level of autonomic activity. The therapist needs to gear such behavioral assignments to the patient's interests and level of motivation.

Some abusing spouses reveal the competitiveness, time urgency, and obsession with achievement commonly associated with the Type A cardiac-prone personality. Such individuals rarely engage in activities that are purely pleasurable without experiencing guilt or agitation. In working toward even small life style changes for the "workaholic" patient, the therapist will inevitably need to elicit and modify cognitions regarding self-worth, achievement, responsibility, and so on, by utilizing many of the techniques described previously. It is not uncommon, therefore, for work and career issues to figure prominently in the treatment of a violent marriage, as the following example illustrates.

An abusing spouse worked long hours as a plumber for a general building contractor. He moonlighted on weekends for extra income, and spent what little time he had left on the endless renovation of the family home. He had long ago forsaken several activities he had loved, most notably camping and fishing in the wilderness. On his job, he described himself as overworked and underpaid, but considered himself lucky to be employed, since he had once been out of work for nearly 3 years. His greatest fear was that if he spoke up for himself at work, he would again find himself without a job. At times he would think, "What's the point of this? I'm living just to go to work every morning." Meanwhile, he rarely verbalized his work-related concerns at home, but would simply behave in a belligerent manner with his wife and children.

At the therapist's urging, the man resumed his outdoor activities, alone at first and later with other members of his family. Predictably, he initially experienced guilt over his fishing expeditions, but quickly learned to relax and enjoy himself. He gradually recognized the connection between his job frustrations and some of the angry interactions in the home. He rarely, if ever, refused the demands of his boss, despite the fact that he seemed to be indispensable to the company. He stated, "I feel as if I ask for a raise or give any less than 125%, I'm taking advantage of the situation." As the man began to discuss his work issues at home, conflict in the family diminished considerably. Moreover, the wife was able to express her support of his position and her esteem for his abilities. He slowly became more realistic in the amount of responsibility he assumed at work, and experienced a considerable drop in tension as he did so. To his surprise, the only thing his boss said when he finally asked for a long overdue raise was, "Okay."

FINAL NOTE

The preceding remarks barely do justice to the complexities of treating violent marriages. The range of cognitive and relationship interventions applicable to such marriages is limited only by the creative potential of the therapist. If this presentation has stimulated further questions, interests, and inventiveness on the part of the reader, then it will have been successful.

REFERENCES

Aponte, H., & Van Deusen, J. Structural family therapy. In A. Gurman & D. Kniskern (Eds.), *Handbook of family therapy*. New York: Brunner/Mazel, 1981.

Beck, A.T. *Cognitive therapy and the emotional disorders*. New York: International Universities Press, 1976.

Beck, A.T. *Cognitive aspects of marital conflict*. Paper presented at the Annual Convention for the Association for the Advancement of Behavior Therapy, New York, 1980.

Beck, A.T., Rush, A.J., Shaw, B.F., & Emery, G. *Cognitive therapy of depression* New York: Guilford Press, 1979.

Bedrosian, R.C. Ecological factors in cognitive therapy: The use of significant others. In G. Emery, S. Hollon, & R. Bedrosian (Eds.), *New directions in cognitive therapy*. New York: Guilford Press, 1981.

Bedrosian, R.C., & Beck, A.T. Principles of cognitive therapy. In M.J. Mahoney (Ed.), *Psychotherapy process: Current issues and future directions*. New York: Plenum Press, 1980.

Coleman, R. Cognitive therapy of agoraphobia. In G. Emery, S. Hollon, & R. Bedrosian (Eds.), *New directions in cognitive therapy*. New York: Guilford Press, 1981.

Emery, G., Hollon, S., & Bedrosian, R. (Eds.). *New directions in cognitive therapy*. New York: Guilford Press, 1981.

Haley, J. *Strategies of psychotherapy*. New York: Grune & Stratton, 1963.

Haley, J. *Problem solving therapy*. San Francisco: Jossey-Bass, 1976.

Hollon, S., Beck, A.T., Bedrosian, R.C., & Young, J. *Combined cognitive-pharmacotherapy versus cognitive therapy in the treatment of depression*. Paper presented at the Annual Meeting of the Society for Psychotherapy Research, Oxford, England, 1979.

Kendall, P., & Hollon, S. (Eds.). *Cognitive-behavioral interventions: Theory, research and procedures*. New York: Academic Press, 1979.

Ledwidge, B. Cognitive behavior modification: A step in the wrong direction? *Psychological Bulletin*, 1978, *85*, 353–375.

Minuchin, S. *Families and family therapy*. Cambridge, Mass.: Harvard University Press, 1974.

Novaco, R. Treatment of chronic anger through cognitive and relaxation controls. *Journal of Consulting and Clinical Psychology*, 1976, *44*, 681.

Novaco, R.W. Anger and coping with stress. In J. Foreyt & D. Rathjen (Eds.), *Cognitive behavior therapy: Research and application*. New York: Plenum Press, 1978.

Rush, A.J., Beck A.T., Kovacs, M., & Hollon, S. Comparative efficacy of cognitive therapy and pharmacotherapy in the treatment of depressed outpatients. *Cognitive Therapy and Research*, 1977, *1*, 17–37.

Watzlawick, P., Beavin, J., & Jackson, D. *Pragmatics of human communication*. New York: Norton, 1967.

9. Beyond Isolated Treatment: A Case for Community Involvement in Family Violence Interventions*

*This article is part of a demonstration program for child abuse and neglect service improvement supported by a grant from the U.S. Department of Health and Human Services, Office of Child Development, National Center on Child Abuse and Neglect (90-CA-870).

Gwen Berghorn, ACSW
Supervisor
Child Abuse Service

Director
Unified Services Project
South Central Community Mental Health Center
Bloomington, Indiana

Anthony Siracusa, M.S.
Clinical Team Leader
Child Abuse Service
South Central Community Mental Health Center
Bloomington, Indiana

Nine

THE INDIVIDUAL THERAPIST WHO ATTEMPTS TO TREAT FAMILY violence without community involvement encounters the following problems:

- a lack of intra-agency peer and supervisory support
- no provision for interagency case or service coordination
- a lack of outreach service to clients
- a community where social agencies do not value others' intervention approaches ("turfism")

This article addresses each of the above problems, providing both theoretical and practical discussion. The goal of the authors is to provide a model for optimum use of inter- and intra-agency support for the individual therapist in the clinical treatment of family violence.

Despite a growing body of knowledge on family violence causes and interventions (Parke & Collmer, 1975), the mental health professions have been slow to respond to the need for treatment. There appear to be multiple reasons to explain this phenomenon; a historical one follows with others addressed in a later section. Early research in the 1960s attributed causality to individual psychosis or personality disorders (Gelles, 1978; Kempe, Silverman, Steele, Droegemuller, & Silver, 1962; Schultz, 1960). Although this unilateral view of the etiology of violence provided license for psychotherapeutic intervention, we suspect, based on our experience and the tendency for therapists to follow the isolated model presented above, that such treatment was often unsuccessful for therapist and client alike. Threads of this historical era remain in psychotherapeutic circles today. A scathing account based primarily on the research of the 1960s and early 70s and written from a feminist viewpoint is presented in Dobash and Dobash (1979).

David Gil (1970) explored the multidimensional aspects underlying the child abuse form of family violence and opened doors for the significant work done in the latter half of the decade by Murray Straus (1977-1978), Justice and Justice (1976), Gelles (1976, 1978), and others. These multidimensional models include social and familial structural causation with roots in psychodynamic theory, cultural norms, and sexual inequality. Justice and Justice (1976), Barnhill (1980), and Helfer and Kempe (1976) have made particularly useful contributions to the application of knowledge to treatment delivery. Also useful to the treatment of family violence is the growing understanding and use of family treatment modalities (Bowen, 1966; Minuchin, 1974; Haley, 1976). The Justices and Barnhill bring the two bodies of knowledge together by illustrating various approaches to working with this population. More recent trends show the development of a cognitive-learning approach (Mahoney, 1977), which Otto and Smith (1980) have applied to child-abuse intervention.

It has now been some 20 years since Henry Kempe began the movement to intervene in family violence by exposing child abuse to a world able to listen. We know enough about causality to justify intervention. We believe it is time the mental health professions respond with some vigor.

THE INTERAGENCY COMMUNITY: SERVICE COORDINATION

Since the causes of family violence are frequently multidimensional, treatment must involve many elements and resources of the community. Child advocates have, for years, proclaimed child abuse to be a community problem (Helfer & Kempe, 1976). Familial violence belongs to the community at large because it strikes at the core of the social structure—its families. The community suffers the effects of battered people in several ways. Those who become socially, emotionally, and physically disabled often lose the ability to produce. Taxpayers bear the cost of remediation and/or maintenance. Certain community institutions feel the effects more than others because of (1) their own efforts at case finding and the ability to provide treatment (social services); (2) legal mandate to intervene; or (3) the availability of resources that provide basic life needs such as food, police protection, shelter, job training and/or employment, day care, education, or "relief from social isolation" (Barnhill, Bloomgarden, Berghorn, Squires, & Siracusa, 1980). Of course, no one agency or service system has all of the resources to deal with all aspects of the family violence problem. The more systems involved and working together, the more comprehensive and cost effective the common response to family violence.

A community system to treat family violence, like any system, must be worked on to be brought into balance and must be nurtured to be maintained. In the beginning the agency price is frustration, stress, and confusion. Later the rewards are positive public relations, interprofessional support, significant contribution to client families, an improved treatment program, and staff with additional skills. The cases often need multiple services over an extended period of time to intervene in the family system. There are seldom enough services in any one geographic area to target all of these problems. Therefore, existing services must be maximized and each agency must play a significant role.

All fifty states have adopted legislation mandating child-protection agencies (and in some states their selected contractors) to investigate and assess reported cases of child abuse and provide services to confirmed cases. Few states have provided similar services to families in which other types of violence occur. Few states and counties have provided mandated agencies with the fiscal resources and number of staff to provide the required interventions. Therefore, even in the child abuse area where resources are state prescribed, interagency support is necessary if adequate interventions are to take place to create change. We have found that, when applicable, effective interagency cooperation is built most successfully in the name of support for those agencies having *legal mandates.*

Provision of services to families in support of and in cooperation with other community agencies means that a mental health facility will not have complete therapeutic control of its clients. It is often difficult to define an agency's role and carry out those and only those services that the agency does best. A community council consisting of agencies and organizations that are in a position to identify and intervene in cases of family violence may be the most efficient entity to coordinate the needs of families, available services, and the roles and responsibilities of each member agency. The size of the geographic community and the number of available services might be allowed to dictate how many councils could be formed. A large city might have one for each family violence area (i.e., child abuse, spouse abuse, and abuse of the elderly and infirm). One council may adequately serve an entire rural county.

Such councils tend to be multifunctional. They provide a forum to air differences and build understanding of each agency's capabilities and limitations. They provide ongoing informal needs assessment and a group to set priorities and develop services to meet the community needs. The council presents a united front for advocacy efforts and community education. When needed, the pooled resources of each agency and the social/political/professional networks of council members can provide a stronger power base than a single agency or individual could develop. Coordination and cooperation can also affect service costs in the community by eliminating or limiting duplication of services. Efficient service delivery is an increasingly important issue. Another important advantage is that through formal training workshops and informal sharing of different disciplinary views, a valuable common knowledge base is acquired.

The interservice council represents an organization that can be effective in primary prevention areas of family violence. Primary prevention services are defined as those which all persons can use and which promote positive family interrelationships. Primary prevention programs provide:

- information about violence and where to receive help
- stress workshops
- cooperative neighborhood day care centers
- parent education
- respite care
- parent-infant services
- volunteer home visitors for the elderly

For practical reasons we recommend that a community service coordinating council be separate from multidisciplinary case planning and disposition teams. (Such a team is discussed below.) Some overlap of the two groups' activities and membership may occur. Each organization has a specific goal, however, and their members often do not have time or energy to do an adequate job on both tasks.

USE OF THE COMMUNITY AT LARGE

Resources outside the intraprofessional and intersocial services systems also provide support for the community response to family violence

(Straus, 1973; Jenkins, MacDicken , & Ormsby, 1979). Obviously, the more people involved, the more comprehensive the community understanding and sense of responsibility for the problem.

Most closely related to the professional intervention system is a paraprofessional and voluntary response. Individuals filling these slots usually do not have any formal training in any particular discipline, but they do have a keen sense of community. Outreach services are very important to mental health agency family violence services and these positions are most often offered to paraprofessionals. While we recommend that occasional home visits be made by primary therapists, regular use of this staff for outreach is generally not cost effective. Outreach workers do a great many of our home assessments and home visits (particularly to clients identified as being at high risk for violence, such as teen parents). They also do a remarkable job in locating resources to fulfill client basic needs and helping clients make best use of such resources. They run many of our family violence primary prevention services such as parent education, assertiveness training, and employment preparation groups. In addition, the outreach worker in our Child Abuse Service manages the entire (volunteer) Parent Aide Program.

Unpaid volunteers are crucial to programming. They become the parent aide corps, run Parents Anonymous meetings, staff the help and hot lines, provide transportation and child care to assist families in coming to therapy sessions, staff women's shelters, provide home emergency shelter, raise money, write and distribute literature, visit the elderly, etc. Volunteers providing direct service to clients can often engage in the client system in a more comprehensive manner than can a therapist or agency outreach worker. They do not represent authority and can put in more time. Therapeutic methods usually offer little beyond group therapy to break a pattern of social isolation. They may be essential, but paraprofessional volunteers offer themselves, their friendship, and often their families as well. Violent families can benefit from both professional and paraprofessional interventions. We find our paraprofessionals often enlighten our assessments, judge well when a family is going into crisis, and provide a fresh outlook on intervention strategies. In this developing field of treatment for family violence, innovation can be most valuable.

Community education campaigns increase understanding of family violence, teach families how and where to receive help, and recruit volunteers. The issue may be kept before the public through professional and paraprofessional speakers addressing service club, church, and special interest groups, printed fliers and brochures, and use of the media. We believe that only through such a campaign can we penetrate the American value system that allows family violence to continue behind closed doors.

Some advice for any publicity on the issues of family violence: (1) keep sensationalism out of your education materials, (2) recognize human feelings and conditions that underlie the problem while rejecting the violent behavioral response, and (3) foster feelings of hope. Sensationalism, righteous indignation, and messages of gloom cause families with the problem to isolate further, further diminish self-esteem, and reduce any hope that their lives can be different. Negative messages tend to recruit volunteers who are angry and want to punish (often they have experienced violence in their own lives) rather than those who are compassionate and want to help. Negative messages also serve to overwhelm the general public and thereby increase acceptance of the problem by fostering its denial.

Broadening community understanding opens other doors as well. Monetary and in-kind donations may be needed to support volunteer recognition, buy play and child-care equipment and library and other educational materials, cover printing and mailing costs, etc. Sites for service delivery, meetings, and training programs are often needed. Churches, libraries, corporate board rooms and training facilities, and service club buildings can all be donated. In 1978 we provided 20 hours of training free to the professional and lay community at a cost of less than $100.00 (Berghorn, Siracusa, & Hitchcock, 1982). A builder in a southwestern state built and donated a women's shelter furnished cooperatively by the community. Costs can be and are shared by many members of the community at large, but they have to understand the problem, feel some concern, be asked, and be publicly recognized for their contribution.

THE INTERPROFESSIONAL COMMUNITY: CASE COORDINATION

Effective service and case coordination are interdependent and enhance one another. Just as one professional in one agency cannot provide all of the services that multiproblem violent families need, one person also often cannot provide adequate intervention to effect change. It has been established that the problems of these families stem from intrapersonal belief systems and poor interpersonal relationship skills. In addition, as

Walker (1977-1978) points out, violence is a family system response to a buildup of frustrations, stress, or threat to one's identity. All family members contribute to the cycles of violent activity and suffer from it. The system itself must have structural features that lock the family into violent response cycles. To complicate the problem further, violent response is learned behavior that may be traced to families of origin (Gayford, 1978; Gelles, 1976). In other words, individuals are socialized to react to certain stimuli by attacking another. The social and cultural demands on the nuclear family make a family member the one most likely to be victimized (Straus, 1977-1978).

If there is a county agency mandated by law to intervene in families on behalf of the victim, that must be the first group of professionals one must work with. It is our experience that they appreciate psychotherapeutic assessment, treatment, and recommendations for many of their clients when we are supportive of their role. In return, they can provide insight into the client from their experience and background. More times than we care to think about, a family's slanted reports of progress in treatment have been countered by a child protection worker's true picture gained from working with the family in the field. It is relatively easy for family members to tell us what they think the therapist wants to hear and play the therapy game in our office. Therefore, the input gained from a colleague in another agency helps us treat the family system as it is rather than from one narrow vantage point. Physicians, educators, school and hospital social workers, public health nurses, and lay volunteers can and do provide real assistance to case management and treatment as well.

Although there is a clear function for the family psychotherapist, therapists tend to avoid treating family violence for three reasons. These are (1) the possibility of a breach of confidentiality, (2) unwillingness to treat persons who may not be self-motivated to change, and (3) reluctance to spend time appearing in court. We are most familiar with the patient-therapist confidentiality issue in the area of child abuse and neglect. This area is also the most pertinent because all fifty states have enacted a version of a mandatory reporting statute that requires mental health professionals to report suspected cases of child abuse and neglect to a mandated investigatory agency. Melvin Guyer (1982) does an excellent job of addressing the clinical and ethical dilemmas faced by mental health professionals in this situation. He concludes that legal requirements may come before patient-therapist confidentiality in the interest of protecting a child.

Our policy is to manage ethical and confidentiality issues by reporting a case in the presence of the family. We explain to the client that we are required by law to do so and we offer support throughout any repercussions such a report might have. Our child protection agency is willing to forgo investigating our reported cases if (1) a release of confidentiality form has been signed to allow interagency communication, (2) the family stays in treatment until the child is no longer at risk, and (3) the child is kept safe from further harm. We have never experienced the loss of a client or further harm to a child as a result of our having reported a case. Families seem more willing to sign releases of information because we support the right not to sign. We also point out that a refusal to sign will hinder us from sharing the family's progress with the authorities. Releases to a variety of agencies are usually signed to incorporate their help and support for the family. Thus, the reporting process is done in a therapeutic manner, helping the family view the therapist as a person in charge who is understanding and supportive. This lessens the fear and provides the family with hope for change.

The second issue that therapists find difficult is treating people who are ordered into therapy by some outside authority, as is often the case with violent families. The situation complicates treatment but need not make it impossible. Violent families often come into therapy threatened and angered by a perception that they are being labeled as ''crazy'' (which also is often their secret belief and their worst fear). In addition, their family systems tend to be rigid (Barnhill, 1979; Barnhill et al.,1980), and such families tend to feel highly threatened by the prospect of change (though also desperately desirous of it). Also, violent clients sometimes enter and stay in treatment only to avoid a worse punishment (they often view treatment as a form of punishment and their weekly visits as ''doing time''—much like a jail sentence).

Most of these problems can be overcome by ''joining'' with the clients. Their ideas, fears, and resistance are eased by showing genuine empathy for their having to do something they don't want to do, acknowledging their right to anger, encouraging their use of the legal system in their behalf, providing a sociostructural explanation of violence rather than a psychological one and working from this model, and assuring them that you expect change to be slow (though nonviolent). A child abuse therapist on our staff points out that he, too, is being ''forced'' by the authorities to treat the family. He reasons that since he and the family are in the situation together, they had better work hard to get the authorities off of all their backs. The client response is usually surprised and positive. A treatment contract with clear goal statements broken down into relatively easy steps to reinforce success is the best way we have found to counteract the ''doing time'' mind set (Justice & Justice, 1976). It is usually helpful if these goals are negotiated in a case conference with the primary helping agencies and the client family represented.

Court-related issues are the third primary reason why mental health professionals shy away from treatment of family violence. The adversarial basis of the judicial system and the social therapeutic system are not designed to work well together. Attorneys and judges determine right and wrong; therapists are often more concerned with helping the parties in opposition—no matter who is right. Therapists bring strong feelings for their clients, their points of view, and their professional integrity into the courtroom only to have all three maligned in the adversarial process. All of this often takes place while the wheels of justice move so slowly that client schedules are disrupted for weeks. If the therapist is in private practice the time factor can represent a severe personal financial burden as well.

Although the situation cannot be changed completely, it can be alleviated in most courts. Some lawyers are willing to sit in on case conferences and some judges are willing to serve on service coordination committees. Others readily agree to go to lunch and be educated about family violence and the therapeutic response while educating you about the legal system in your community. Bringing the prosecutor into your agency to talk at an inservice training and to hear your views can be a powerful bridge between the two systems. Judges can often be reasoned with to take a deposition in chambers at a mutually convenient time. Others will have a clerk phone you just prior to the time you will take the stand so that you need not wait at the courthouse. Educating judges about the services you offer and how to make appropriate court-ordered referrals can also facilitate coordination of the two systems.

INTRA-AGENCY DEVELOPMENT: THE INTRA-AGENCY COMMUNITY

Mental health agencies will benefit from working with other community agencies but it will not be enough. They also must learn to adapt their own policies and procedures to treat violent family clients. Different types of abuse also must be treated somewhat differently though their etiologies are in many ways similar. (See Barnhill et al., 1980; Straus, 1977-1978; Rathbone-McCuan, 1980, for comparison.) Because of the difficulty in treating families prone to violence, administrative sanction is often an important step. There needs to be a willingness to evaluate across the agency and consider small changes in procedures to facilitate treatment.

Families who become violent tend to seek help only when in crises and then tend not to follow through. Requests for help usually follow such subtle patterns as identifying other presenting problems, showing up at hospital emergency rooms with elaborate fabrications of how injuries came about, or acting out in the community.

Both victims and perpetrators tend to label themselves as "bad" either because they inflict injury or because they believe they deserve it. They typically find it difficult to trust authorities for fear of having their self-views confirmed or being told they are in some way inadequate. Self-righteousness is often portrayed and sometimes is a part of the client's belief system. Clients miss scheduled appointments, are often hostile, recalcitrant, usually highly manipulative, and generally highly unresponsive to traditional agency methods of service delivery. Both the therapist and the agency must adapt new methods to deal with the situation. Dr. John Reinhart is quoted in *Child Abuse and Neglect: The Problem and its Management* (U.S. Department of Health, Education and Welfare, 1975). "You've got to go out to (these people) . . . Therapists . . . often have to modify their practice by occasionally seeing parents at home, chasing them down the hallway, and seeing them at odd times—like two weeks late. Every system has to learn . . . modifications of traditional resources and procedures" (p. 66). Trust is slow to develop among these clients. And the initial stages of treatment can take several months.

A second step for developing services for this population is training therapists to make modifications in their treatment methods for more effective planning and outcome. For purposes of intra-agency service coordination and referral, all staff should receive some training. If no one in the agency has a developed specialty in this area, contracting for ongoing outside program consultation and case supervision may be valuable in the beginning stages of the program. Family violence treatment is difficult, and good training, supervision, and peer support systems will prevent staff burnout.

The third crucial step is an inhouse evaluation and coordination across the system. This step can be relatively informal but it should be thorough. The crisis/emergency staff should know how to identify a case, special ways of dealing with it so that treatment begins immediately, what is required of them by state law, and how to go about it without further alienating the client(s). Intake procedures may need to be modified so that clients receive treatment as soon as possible following referral. Policies for missed appointments may need to be reassessed. Who pays for court-ordered services? Will family treatment be offered or will parents see one therapist in one department and children be required to seek treatment elsewhere? Coordination with addiction specialists may be very important. How are clients identified and assigned to appropriate services/therapists? Diagnosis for treatment and for third-party payments may be an issue.

The final inhouse activity is reaching out both to other community agencies (if this is not already in process) and to client families. Educating the community is similar to marketing your product. Campaigns to reach clients must be compassionate and must indicate a nonjudgmental approach to violence. (''All parents feel like hitting their children at times and all children need discipline—if you are afraid that you'll go too far and feel sorry afterward give us a call''—or something similar to reach the target client population.) Even if other community agencies are responding negatively to your offer of services, we advise that case finding activities continue. The resulting community tension will act as a catalyst to bring about changes and new balance in the community care-giving system.

A MULTIDISCIPLINARY DIAGNOSTIC/TREATMENT TEAM APPROACH

The idea of having different agencies meet to discuss a case is not new. It has happened for years, but has been reserved by community caregivers for situations that were especially difficult and cases that appeared impossible to treat. As we have mentioned, the families who are typically involved in violence can be characterized by their multiple problems and the chronicity of this behavior. Therapists and other human service professionals often find themselves alone when treating these families. They infrequently call on the unique support system that can be found among other human service professionals within their community, and in this respect they suffer from the same self-imposed isolation as the troubled families they treat.

Our experience has been in treating the child-abusing family. We will use this as our model for relating the team approach to breaking the isolation of family violence treatment. The team concept for treating abuse is about 25 years old and was originally hospital based (Kempe, 1978). Team membership was composed of a medical social worker, a pediatrician, and a nurse. Community-based treatment teams, which are often called child protection teams, are generally under the leadership of the Department of Public Welfare. These teams formulate their decision making from the broader base of the child welfare system and the Department of Public Welfare's interface with the court.

Many communities have neither, and in 1978 ours was no exception. As mental health professionals, we found ourselves with a number of cases that were resistant to almost any intervention. In the face of frustration and stress, individual therapists began meeting regularly to discuss abusive client families. Eventually, with a push from the Department of Public Welfare, in the form of a plea for assistance, our administrators supported clinicians, child protection workers, and other involved community professionals in forming a treatment team. This mental-health-based team has evolved over the last four years. Below we describe the key elements of this approach

Team Purpose

The overall purpose of the mental-health-based team is to assess, diagnose, and treat all members of the violent family from a coordinated interagency perspective. As family therapists we adhere to a systemic approach and recognize not only the influence of family members, but community caregivers as well. For example, abusive families are frequently ordered into treatment by the court or under the watchful eye of the Department of Public Welfare. Now the family problem includes not only the abuse, but the public agency that has control over the custody of the child. As Haley (1976) notes, ''when social control is an issue, the professional milieu is part of the presenting problem'' (p. 3).

However, working as a collective, community caregivers have minimized problems and allowed members to realize some of the specific purposes of the team:

1. Providing community networking between agencies so a comprehensive approach is taken for dealing with family dysfunction.

2. Having a greater data base through professional input to allow for better diagnostic and treatment disposition decisions on new cases.
3. Maintaining a peer support system to address the emotionally draining aspect of this work and to counter ''burnout.''
4. Reviewing cases through peer supervision thereby promoting the concept of shared responsibility and guarding against unilateral decisionmaking, which may adversely affect a family.
5. Identifying weaknesses in our system that may be more readily pinpointed by other community caregivers.

Team Membership and Roles

Members are placed on the team according to certain functions that need to be performed and treatment issues that must be addressed. For dealing with cases of child abuse in a mental health setting we chose to have clinicians from several different service areas. The service areas and personnel are:

Mental-Health-Center-Based Members

1. Child Abuse Services
Team Leader. Coordinates the implementation of team recommendations and consults with other team members on clinical issues of an emergent nature.
Child Abuse Specialist. Functions as a generalist in treating all forms of child abuse and working with the community.
Outreach Worker. Performs home assessments and also supervises volunteer parent aides.
Child Treatment Specialists. Three clinicians who are part of a federally funded program to provide mental health services to abused children.
2. Children and Youth Services. Two psychologists who evaluate children and do custody evaluations.
3. Addictions Services. A substance abuse specialist.
4. Adult Outpatient Services. A psychiatric social worker with expertise for working in the area of spouse abuse.

These clinicians all have solid therapy skills and use them in conjunction with the special services they provide families. In many instances, team members act as cotherapists when the different expertise of two therapists is needed, or when a case presents itself as so unmanageable that the support of another therapist appears appropriate. When two therapists work together, one is always designated primary therapist or case manager.

Community-Based Members

1. Department of Public Welfare. Three child protection workers are the source of referrals for more than 54% of the team cases (additional referral sources include "self" referrals, and other social agencies).
2. Public Health Nurse. A public health nurse provides the team with medical input on cases.
3. Other involved community personnel are invited to attend disposition and review meetings for cases they are servicing. Release of information forms signed by the clients must include all personnel.

Diagnosis and Service Planning

From either a scheduled intake or an emergency service contact, all cases of child abuse and neglect are presented to the multidisciplinary diagnostic/treatment team by the person who did the intake. The team meets weekly for 1 hour. New cases are presented first, and the remaining time is spent on cases members wish to review. Once a month the team has a 2-hour meeting to work on administrative agenda or receive inservice training.

Present at each meeting are regular team members and any "invited" referring professionals. The team processes about three new cases a month and reviews about ten cases each week. The same case may be reviewed several weeks in a row especially if it is problematic to team caregivers. As we mentioned, families referred for abuse are multiproblem, and a problem-oriented record (POR) is utilized. Similar to the instrument developed by Schmitt (1978), the POR allows for the development of an active problem list that cuts across basic life domains of all family members. The POR helps us identify the areas of stress on the family and plan comprehensive management and intervention strategies. It is with the collaboration of the involved professionals, and the careful documentation of family problem areas, that an initial disposition is arrived at. In addition, the process provides the basis for a clear, goal-oriented treatment contract to be developed with the family.

Review of a case can be requested by any team member working on that case, or the team leader. This process usually incorporates input on how the family is doing in treatment, and how it is functioning in the community. Reviews often result in interagency plans to work more effectively with the family.

CONCLUSIONS

The therapist who faces the treatment of the violent family alone is likely to find himself or herself shouldering a stressful burden. There are often high-intensity emotions that challenge the therapist working with the violent family, and these may hinder appropriate management and treatment decisions.

Presented here is a model of developing resources both within and between community agencies and professional groups that can provide support for the therapist in treating this difficult population. There are several implications for treating families with this approach. Since there are multiple factors leading to the violence in these families, the more comprehensive the approach, the less likely it is that something will be missed that may provide a catalyst for the next violent episode. By having a larger and tighter "net," the families who might "fall through the cracks" are brought to our attention by better case finding. Our regular team meetings provide greater service delivery continuity because therapists are aware of evolving family circumstances. Finally, when responsibility is shared by several professionals no one person feels as vulnerable to making a wrong decision.

The treatment of violence in families is still a psychotherapy area undergoing rapid development. The community and agency programs discussed here have taken four years to develop. A similar thrust would take a great amount of work as well as careful planning and time. However, the rewards of more effective service to an especially hard to reach population and personal benefits for therapists should be substantial.

REFERENCES

Barnhill, L., Healthy family systems. *Family Coordinator*, 1979, *28*, 94–100.
Barnhill, L. Clinical assessment of intra-familial violence. *Hospital and Community Psychiatry*, 1980, *31*, 543–547.

Barnhill, L., Bloomgarden, R., Berghorn, G., Squires, M., & Siracusa, A. Clinical and community interventions in violence in families. In L. Wolberg & M. Aronson, *Group and family therapy: 1980.* New York: Brunner/Mazel, 1980.

Berghorn, G.L., Siracusa, A.J., & Hitchcock, R.A. Development of a training program for treatment providers in child abuse and neglect cases. *Proceedings of the Fourth National Conference on Child Abuse and Neglect,* Los Angeles, California, October 1982.

Bowen, M. The use of family theory in clinical practice. *Comprehensive Psychiatry,* 1966, *7,* 345–374.

Dobash, E., & Dobash, R. *Violence against wives.* New York: Free Press, 1979.

Gayford, J.J. Battered wives. In J.P. Martin (Ed.), *Violence and the family.* New York: Wiley, 1978.

Gelles, R.J. Abused wives: Why do they stay? *Journal of Marriage and the Family,* 1976, *38,* 659–668.

Gelles, R.J. Violence in the American family. In J.P. Martin (Ed.), *Violence and the family.* New York: Wiley, 1978.

Gil, D.G. *Violence against children: Physical child abuse in the United States.* Cambridge, Mass.: Harvard University Press, 1970.

Guyer, M.J. Child abuse and neglect statutes: Legal and clinical implications. *American Journal of Orthopsychiatry,* 1982, *52,* 73–81.

Haley, J. *Problem-solving therapy.* San Francisco: Jossey-Bass, 1976.

Helfer, R., & Kempe, C. *Child abuse and neglect: The family and the community.* Cambridge, Mass.: Ballinger, 1976.

Jenkins, J.L., MacDicken, R.A., & Ormsby, N.J. *A community approach: The child protection coordinating committee* (U.S. Department of Health, Education and Welfare, DHEW Pub. No. [OHDS] 79-30195). Washington, D.C.: Government Printing Office, 1979.

Justice, B., & Justice R. *The abusing family.* New York: Human Sciences Press, 1976.

Kempe, H. Foreword. In Schmitt, B. (Ed.), *The child protection handbook.* New York: Garland STPM Press, 1978.

Kempe, C.H., Silverman, F., Steele, B.F., Droegemuller, W., & Silver, H.K. The battered child syndrome. *Journal of the American Medical Association,* 1962, *181,* 17–24.

Mahoney, M.J. Reflections on the cognitive-learning trend in psychotherapy. *American Psychologist,* 1977, *1,* 5–13.

Minuchin, S. *Families and family therapy.* Cambridge, Mass.: Harvard University Press, 1974.

Otto, M.L., & Smith, D.G. Child abuse: A cognitive behavioral intervention model. *Journal of Marital and Family Therapy,* 1980, *8,* 425–429.

Parke, R.D., & Collmer, C.W. Child abuse: An interdisciplinary analysis, In E.M. Hetherington (Ed.), *Review of child development research* (Vol. 5). Chicago: University of Chicago Press, 1975.

Rathbone-McCuan, E. Elderly victims of family violence and neglect. *Social Casework,* 1980, *25,* 296–304.

Schmitt, B. (Ed.). *The child protection handbook.* New York: Garland STPM Press, 1978.

Schultz, L. The wife assaulter. *Journal of Social Therapy,* 1960, *6,* 103–112.

Straus, M.A. A general systems theory approach to a theory of violence between family members. *Social Science Information,* 1973, *12,* 105–123.

Straus, M.A. Wife beating: How common and why? *Victimology*, 1977-1978, *3/4*, 443-457.

U.S. Department of Health, Education and Welfare. *Child abuse and neglect: The problem and its management* Vol. 31 *The community team: An approach to case management and prevention.* (OHD, OCD, Children's Bureau, NCCAN, DHEW Publ. No. [OHD] 75-30075). Washington, D.C.: Government Printing Office, 1975.

Walker, L. Battered women and learned helplessness. *Victimology*, 1977-1978, *3/4*, 532.